Physical Examination
of the Newborn
at a Glance

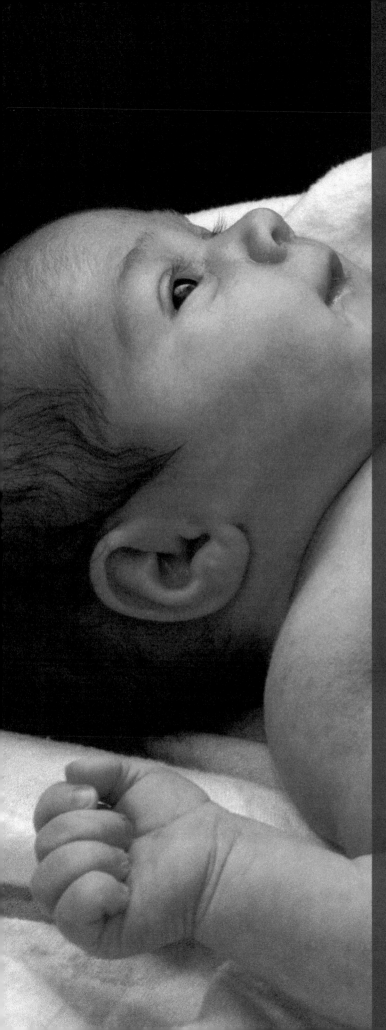

Physical Examination of the Newborn
at a Glance

Denise (Dee) Campbell

RN, RM, BSc, PgDip, MA, FHEA
Principal Lecturer and Programme Tutor in
Midwifery (*retired*)
University of Hertfordshire
Hatfield, UK

Lyn Dolby

RN, RM, MSc, FHEA
Senior Lecturer and Programme Leader in
Midwifery
University of Northampton
Northampton, UK

Series Editor

Ian Peate OBE, FRCN

WILEY Blackwell

This edition first published 2018
© 2018 John Wiley & Sons Ltd.

The right of Denise Campbell and Lyn Dolby to be identified as the authors of this work has been asserted in accordance with law.

Registered Offices
John Wiley & Sons, Inc., 111 River Street, Hoboken, NJ 07030, USA
John Wiley & Sons Ltd., The Atrium, Southern Gate, Chichester, West Sussex, PO19 8SQ, UK

Editorial Office
9600 Garsington Road, Oxford, OX4 2DQ, UK

For details of our global editorial offices, customer services, and more information about Wiley products visit us at www.wiley.com.

Wiley also publishes its books in a variety of electronic formats and by print-on-demand. Some content that appears in standard print versions of this book may not be available in other formats.

Library of Congress Cataloging-in-Publication Data are available

ISBN: 9781119155577

Cover image: © chameleonseye/Gettyimages
Cover design by Wiley

Set in Minion Pro 9.5/11.5 pt by Aptara
Printed and bound by CPI Group (UK) Ltd, Croydon, CR0 4YY

C9781119155577_230124

Contents

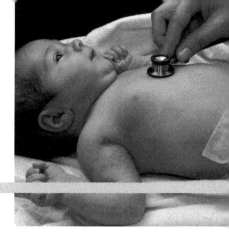

Part 6   Revision and self-assessment   105

Preface

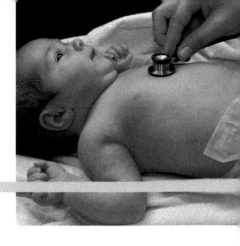

Since the early 1990s, midwives have been able to access further training in order to become Newborn and Infant Physical Examination (NIPE) practitioners and incorporate the examination of the newborn into their daily practice. Not all midwives have yet undertaken the course, but in recent years a growing number of higher education institutions have started to incorporate the course into their pre-registration midwifery programmes. This action not only aligns with one of the key points highlighted within the document *Midwifery 2020* (Department of Health, 2010), but also enables midwifery students to conduct solo NIPEs at the point of registration as a qualified midwife.

However, this book is not for the sole use of midwives or student midwives, as there have been a growing number of neonatal intensive care nurses who also access the course. Therefore, the content of this book seeks to give both students and those already qualified as NIPE practitioners an 'at-a-glance' understanding of the key elements that relate to this valuable skill. For some, this will be the first step in their journey to become NIPE practitioners, for others this book will provide a revision aid or an opportunity to update professional knowledge and understanding.

We strongly believe that the examination is an important part of normal, holistic, woman-centred care. The content of this book covers the main conditions and issues relating to physical examination of the newborn. We have also provided some crosswords and multiple choice questions to enable the reader to undertake a short self-test.

We hope the reader finds this book a useful aid to learning and professional practice.

Reference

Department of Health. (2010). Midwifery 2020: Delivering Expectations. London: The Stationery Office. Retrieved from: https://www.gov.uk/government/uploads/system/uploads/attachment_data/file/216029/dh_119470.pdf (accessed 23 October 2017).

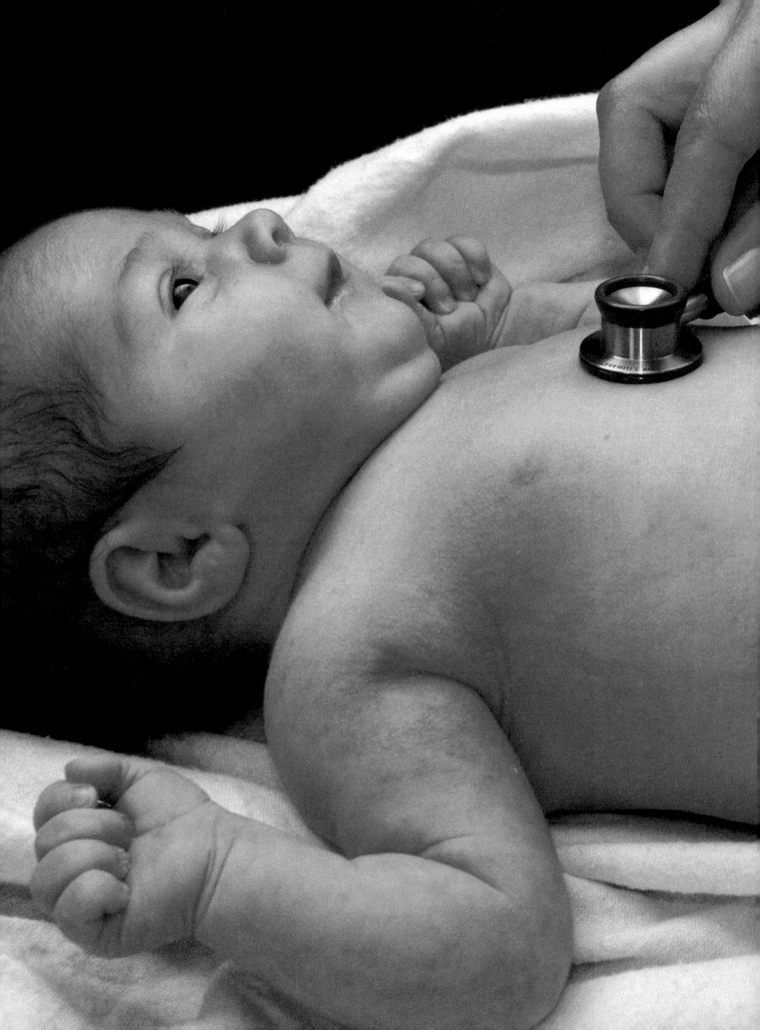

Professional issues

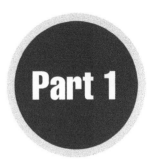

Part 1

Chapters

1 Public health screening

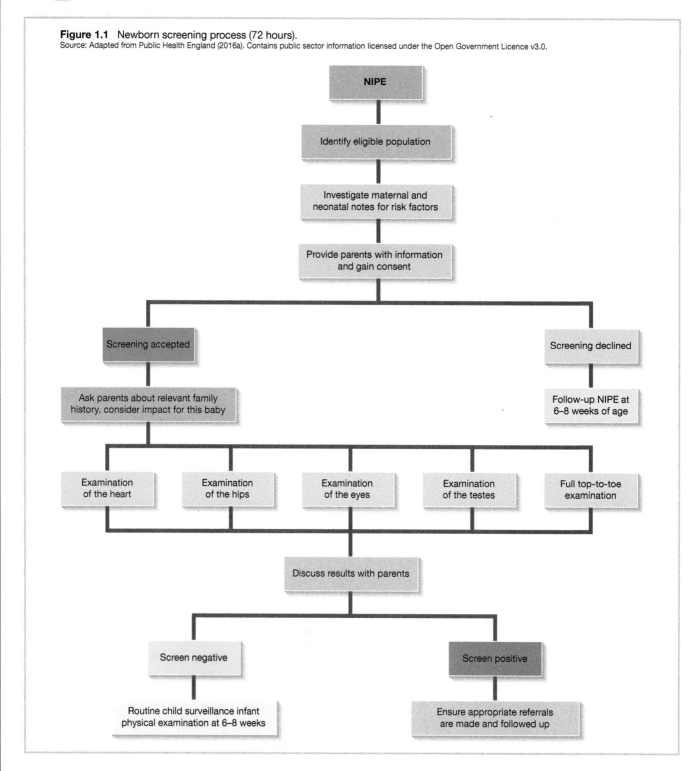

Figure 1.1 Newborn screening process (72 hours).
Source: Adapted from Public Health England (2016a). Contains public sector information licensed under the Open Government Licence v3.0.

Public Health England (PHE) is an operationally autonomous executive agency of the Department of Health. The prime role of PHE is to reduce health inequality and protect and improve the health and well-being of the nation's individuals. The National Health Service (NHS) national population screening programmes are developed and implemented on the advice given by the National Screening Committee (NSC) in the United Kingdon (UK). The NSC provides evidence-based recommendations to government ministers in all four UK countries.

PHE supports its activities by drawing evidence from world class research and by promoting advocacy and collaborative partnerships, all of which assist the delivery of specialist public

Physical Examination of the Newborn at a Glance, First Edition. Denise (Dee) Campbell and Lyn Dolby.
© 2018 John Wiley & Sons, Ltd. Published 2018 by John Wiley & Sons, Ltd.

health services. It is also in close liaison with the Screening Quality Assurance Service who, by investigating whether national standards are met, can verify if screening programmes are safe and effective. In relation to the NHS Newborn and Infant Physical Examination (NIPE) Screening Programme, both the *NIPE Handbook 2016/2017* and the *NIPE Screening Programme Standards 2016/2017* were published to inform and support best clinical practice. These texts will subsequently be updated and amended to reflect the available evidence and therefore it is important that practitioners refer to the latest edition. It is also important that the Service specification 2016/2017 (No. 21) (Public Health England, 2016a) is also referred to in the same manner.

Screening is not diagnostic

Population screening is a way of identifying healthy people who may be at increased risk of a disease or condition. When an individual is highlighted as being at a higher risk of developing the disease or condition in question, then they can receive further information, investigations or treatment. The provision of screening aims to reduce the risks or complications associated with a disease or condition.

Screening is *not* a diagnostic process. Without further investigation, a screening process cannot usually provide confirmation that an individual has a specific disease or condition. However, newborn blood spot screening does merge these two processes, as screening is offered for all babies so there will be some babies in whom a specific condition is confirmed and so subsequent treatment and management of the condition can be offered.

In relation to NIPE, there are four main screening elements that are assessed: eyes, heart, hips and testes. This is not because examining the baby for other conditions is not important (including a full top-to-toe), but because these four elements can be systematically measured and therefore, standards relating to good practice and timescales can be set accordingly.

NIPE policy

The NSC requires that all eligible babies should be offered the NIPE within 72 hours of birth (Figure 1.1). A second NIPE is offered again at 6–8 weeks of age by the family's general practitioner (GP). However, it is the responsibility of the birth unit to identify all eligible babies (including those who move into the area), which will continue until the 72-hour NIPE is completed or responsibility for this is transferred to another acute care provider. The responsibility for following up on referrals after the 6-week examination rests with the GP, who should check the care pathway for progression in relation to referrals or results of action taken.

The main aim of the NIPE programme is to detect any congenital abnormalities of the eyes, heart, hips and testes, where these are detectable within the first 72 hours after birth. The examination at 6–8 weeks provides a second opportunity to detect these abnormalities at the end of the neonatal period. The ending of the neonatal period is when most of the physiological changes that occur after birth have been completed. Most babies will have made the transition from fetal to neonatal life and conditions arising after this time will not necessarily be congenital in origin. However, if an abnormality is undetected or masked by another condition or illness, then it may still be first recognised because of parental concern or because the baby exhibits signs and symptoms of the condition. It is a salient point to note that parental concerns should be taken seriously – they know their child and changes in behaviour or ability will often be clear to them.

Parental information

All parents should be given information relating to the NIPE, in terms of what it is, why it is offered and when it is performed and by whom. During the antenatal period and before the NIPE is conducted, a leaflet and discussion should take place, so that questions can be answered and to give the parents time to think about any family history that the practitioner may not be aware of.

Verbal consent should be obtained from the parents prior to conducting the examination. During the examination, the ability of the baby should be mentioned and any concerns that the parents have should be addressed. The findings of the examination should be discussed with them prior to completing a comprehensive record (see Chapter 3). They should also be informed who to contact if they have concerns about their baby's health and that the second main examination for their baby will be when he/she is 6–8 weeks of age when any queries remaining from the 72-hour NIPE should be addressed. For example, the baby may have had unilateral undescended testes at the 72-hour examination and the parents will need to know if this has now resolved. The documentation should reflect the fact that previous findings have been noted, the findings of the 6–8 week examination plus any further actions that may be required.

Key considerations

NIPE recommends that the 72-hour examination should be undertaken for all babies prior to discharge home. This maximises the likelihood that the examination will be completed in a timely manner. It is also advantageous to the parents, as some will not want to return to the hospital after being discharged home. There will also be some who will choose not to return and not to take part in screening when they are no longer in an environment where it is easily accessed.

If an examination must be performed early in neonatal life when auscultating for heart murmurs is more likely, it is preferential to do so rather than the examination not be conducted and therefore at risk of a heart murmur being missed. As with a baby of any point in the first 72-hours, there is always the possibility of hearing a heart murmur and therefore the information given in relation to signs of ill health is no less or more important for one baby during this time, than any other.

If a baby has been admitted to a neonatal intensive care unit (NICU) or special care baby unit (SCBU), then all practitioners in contact with the baby should ensure that the key elements of the NIPE are assessed when practicable to do so. If a baby has been discharged home from NICU or SCBU, then practitioners in the community such as the midwife, health visitor or GP need to investigate if the NIPE has been comprehensively completed, as sometimes this can be missed.

As with any programme, the completion of its component parts is paramount and NIPE SMART will assist in highlighting errors or omissions. However, the process of completion will still only be as good as the attention to detail of the professionals involved.

2 Quality and standard setting

Figure 2.1 Examination of the newborn (72 hour): standards and guidance.

NIPE Standard 3		
Examination finding	**NIPE descriptor**	**Performance thresholds**
↓	↓	↓
Positive screening test	Percentage of babies who have specialist hip USS within 2 weeks of age	**Acceptable** ≥95% of babies → USS by 2 weeks of age
		Achievable 100% of babies → USS by 2 weeks of age
NIPE Standard 4		
Negative screening test, but positive factor	Percentage of babies who have specialist hip USS within 6 weeks of age	**Acceptable** ≥95% of babies → USS by 2 weeks of age
		Achievable 100% of babies → USS by 2 weeks of age

NIPE, Newborn and Infant Physical Examination; USS, ultrasound screening.

Figure 2.2 Examination of the newborn (6–8 weeks): standards and guidance.

NIPE Standard 3		
Examination finding	**NIPE descriptor**	**Performance thresholds**
↓	↓	↓
Positive screening test	Percentage of babies who are seen by orthopaedic surgeon by 10 weeks of age	**Acceptable** ≥95% of babies → by 10 weeks of age
		Achievable 100% of babies → by 10 weeks of age

Physical Examination of the Newborn at a Glance, First Edition. Denise (Dee) Campbell and Lyn Dolby.
© 2018 John Wiley & Sons, Ltd. Published 2018 by John Wiley & Sons, Ltd.

NHS Trusts utilise a systematic approach to maintain and improve the quality of patient care whilst reducing risk. To achieve these aims, robust processes are put in place to facilitate the audit of areas such as clinical effectiveness, education and training, risk management and transparency in relation to investigation and policy. In effect, quality assurance provides a process that enables continuous audit of progress, standard of practice and/or activity and the identification of issues that require improvement. Quality assurance assists in assessing if the standards set are not only being met, but are also appropriate and feasible.

Each of the NHS national screening programmes has its own clearly defined set of standards. However, in order that the process of quality assurance is robust and comprehensive, several factors should be considered. First, a screening programme is developed and overseen by a committee who have experience and knowledge in that specific field of expertise or who have first-hand knowledge (professionals and service users). The facilitation of a quality review of the service includes diverse participants such as those involved in commissioning or providing screening services as well as those who use the service.

The committee assists in the development of national quality standards. This involves setting up processes that can monitor how the service meets (or not) the standards set. In the event of adverse incidents, the committee also provides access to expert screening advice to allow for effective incident management.

Quality assurance is all-encompassing and covers the screening process from start to finish. This process commences with the premise that the screening programme is justifiable; it decides who will be offered screening; assesses the quality throughout the screening activity and continues through to referral when this is required. In relation to the Newborn and Infant Physiological Examination (NIPE), the main aim is to provide a screening service that is accessible to all women and their babies and that a minimum standard is maintained in order to minimise harm whilst maximising the benefit derived from screening.

A consistent driver within quality assurance is the need to maintain a high-quality service. Collaboration with local screening programmes through involvement of local teams is important. Effective team working necessitates that professionals, commissioners and the screening committee work towards risk reduction and ensure that audit trails are working effectively. A process that works well should be able to respond appropriately to incidents and allow productive inter-professional communication to take place if the issue is to be resolved and to promote the sharing of good practices.

Quality assurance is inevitably a formal process and each local screening programme is responsible for its own effectiveness. This is monitored by statistical review, regional meetings or even informal visits. The NIPE standards give a parameter to work towards, which is feasible and allows for the very slight local differences that occur from region to region.

Key performance indicators

Key performance indicators (KPIs) were introduced into NHS screening programmes to assist in the measurement of performance within specific areas. They act as a tool to govern and assess performance, by helping to identify potential or actual problems. Highlighting issues is important if the root cause is to be uncovered and a solution found to remedy the situation. The NIPE screening programme currently has two KPIs (NP1 and NP2), which can be viewed in the *NIPE Screening Programme Handbook* (Public Health England, 2016a) and the *NIPE Screening Programme Standards 2016/2017* (Public Health England, 2016b).

It is good practice for NHS Trusts to maintain a list of NIPE practitioners to detail when a practitioner qualified, if they conduct NIPEs regularly (this is a Trust, not a Public Health England parameter) and when the practitioner last attended an updating course. No arena of professional practice stands still for long and both the Nursing and Midwifery Council and the General Medical Council require practitioners to update and maintain a high level of professional knowledge and skill as well as recognise when care has not been in keeping with the standards set. The use of the NIPE SMART system enables data to be collected that identify areas of shortfall, near misses or those areas where clinical performance is exemplary. Those Trust sites where NIPE SMART is not yet operational have had to put in place their own methods of auditing the standards.

Figures 2.1 and 2.2 show a visual representation of the standards and guidelines set; in this instance, developmental dysplasia of the hip (DDH) is used as an example. These standards and guidelines reflect the serious consequences for the baby if further investigation or treatment is delayed. In this example, late detection of DDH not only has implications for the baby in terms of discomfort, reduced mobility and the prospect of increasing the level of trauma, but it also highlights the future impact on the individual (see Chapter 44). Woodacre *et al.* (2014) pointed out that the cost of treating DDH early not only clearly reduces the level of impact to the individual, but greatly reduces the cost incurred of treating DDH at a later stage. Treating the condition later often becomes more complex and the need for surgical intervention is higher. The psychological impact on the child and parents can also be higher with later diagnosis.

Therefore, it can be demonstrated that if the available literature points to the need for early treatment to prevent or reduce the impact of a dislocated hip, then it is sensible to assess the available services, in terms of training and referral pathways, as well as produce publications relating to expected professional activity and the standards and guidelines that should reflect best practice.

All NIPE practitioners should keep a record of babies that they have referred in order to check on outcomes. This assists with learning, as it encourages self-reflection in terms of one's knowledge base and awareness of the condition and appropriate referral processes, as well as the discussion that took place with the parents and the accuracy of information given. The standards and guidelines may not appear directly related to such activity, but it is inevitable that professional practice and how it is carried out has a strong part to play in meeting the thresholds set for each NIPE standard.

In relation to the Trust site, the guidelines clearly pinpoint the levels that are considered 'acceptable' and 'achievable'. If these thresholds are not being met, then the Trust is obliged to investigate where the problem lies. For example, it is possible that there are too few experienced NIPE practitioners available to help support those who are newer to the role, or it could be that data are missing. Some issues can be resolved and therefore it is important that they are highlighted. It is important to take into account factors that cannot be easily resolved, at least making the issue known.

3 Record keeping and professional competency

Figure 3.1 Think about your professional role in relation to NIPE and the importance of *your* voice in multi-professional communication.

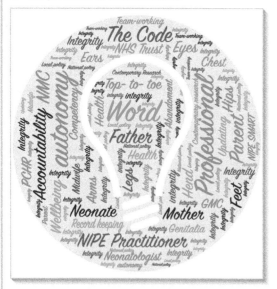

Figure 3.2 The Code.

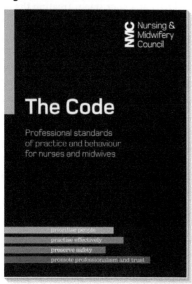

Figure 3.3 The Personal Child Health Record.

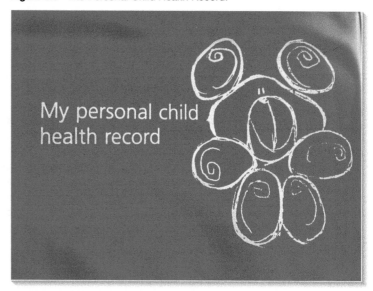

Figure 3.4 NIPE SMART.

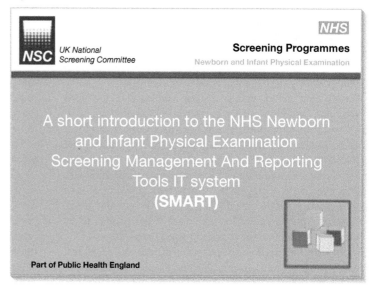

Physical Examination of the Newborn at a Glance, First Edition. Denise (Dee) Campbell and Lyn Dolby.
© 2018 John Wiley & Sons, Ltd. Published 2018 by John Wiley & Sons, Ltd.

Record keeping

Every practitioner is responsible for the record that they make in relation to care or information given, the rationale for action taken and the summarised discussion that occurs between parents and practitioners and between healthcare professionals (Figure 3.1). When completing the appropriate records on the examination of the newborn, the same diligence and attention to detail applies. The findings of the examination and a summary of the salient points of discussion between the parents and the practitioner, including any parental concerns and the reassurance or information given at the time, should be clearly documented.

Parents should always be informed, who else will have access to their child's record, such as paediatricians, health visitors and social workers.

Both the Nursing and Midwifery Council (NMC, 2015) (Figure 3.2) and the General Medical Council (GMC, 2012; Abdelrahman and Abdelmageed, 2014) provide guidance on professional and ethical practice which incorporates the principles of good record keeping. These principles include the following key elements:

- Handwriting should be legible.
- All entries to records must be signed. In the case of written records, most records (including the National Neonatal notes), provide a section to complete with the name of the practitioner (in block capitals) designation and signature. However, if this is absent within the local records, the practitioner's name must be placed alongside his/her signature for ease of identification.
- The date and time should be given for every record entry and this should be in real time and in chronological order. The entry should be made as contemporaneously as possible, being as close to the actual time as would be considered feasible. For example, it should not take 3 hours to commence writing the findings of an examination unless, for example, an emergency occurred, in which case the reason for the delay should be documented in the notes.
- Records should be accurate and recorded in such a way that the meaning is clear, factual and does not include unnecessary abbreviations, jargon, meaningless phrases or irrelevant speculation.
- Professional judgement and local policy will give insight into what information is relevant and what should be recorded.
- Records should provide an accurate summary of activity, findings, discussion and information giving with parent(s) and other healthcare professionals, management plans and actions taken.
- Any alterations or additions should be clearly marked as such, with accompanying date and time and rationale for doing so.
- The parent(s) should be aware of the findings that the practitioner is summarising within the notes and need to understand the language that he/she is using. If necessary, most NHS Trusts have an interpreter service (participants are expected to maintain confidentiality).
- Written records should also be readable in the event that they need to be photocopied or scanned. Therefore, use of a black ink pen is still preferable to any other colour ink.
- Only use an abbreviation that is contained within the local NHS Trust list and never a personal one. This prevents confusion occurring between healthcare professionals.

In general, the records that are completed in relation to the Newborn and Infant Physiological Examination (NIPE) include the local NHS Trust Neonatal Notes and digital record, the Personal Child Health Record (PCHR) and the SMART system which was set up by Public Health England (PHE), National Screening Committee (NSC) to assist in the capture of data relating to the NIPE for audit and failsafe purposes. More information on the failsafe standards can be viewed on the NIPE website.

The PCHR (Figure 3.3) is given to the parents for each child that is born. It is a document that is frequently updated in line with current practice and today's technology. The contemporary version can always be viewed on the Health for All Children website (see useful websites section in the references). The latest updates are highlighted and an explanation given for any changes made. It should also be noted that even with the available digital technology, the paper version of the PCHR is still available in order to allow all parents equal access.

The SMART system (Figure 3.4) has been rolled out across many NHS Trust sites, but to reduce repetition between the Trust's digital records and the SMART system, PHE/NSC are gradually adapting how it captures the information in order that it can do so automatically from the Trust's digital record rather than being populated by the practitioner. This saves time, repetition and reduces error. For further information on SMART see useful websites section in the references.

Professional responsibilities

The NIPE must only be completed by a healthcare professional who has been appropriately trained to provide the duty of care required. The healthcare professionals that can conduct the NIPE include members of the paediatric team, advanced neonatal nurse practitioners, general practitioners, midwives and student midwives working under supervision with a NIPE practitioner (in those areas where there is agreement with the local university).

It should be borne in mind that not all universities include the training for NIPE within the initial pre-registration programme of midwifery, enabling midwifery students to conduct the NIPE at the point of qualification as a midwife. Therefore, NHS Trusts will often require clear evidence that the NIPE qualification has been successfully achieved.

The NIPE programme does not stipulate numbers of NIPEs or what form of updating that NIPE practitioners should undertake in order to maintain their level of competency. However, they suggest that some form of yearly update should be considered, which includes a practical update and annual completion of the NIPE e-learning modules (see useful e-learning resources section in the references). It is good practice to reflect on one's competence and level of expertise and each practitioner should also consider attending an appropriate conference or study day that relates to the aspects of the NIPE.

Although the NIPE programme does not stipulate numbers of NIPEs that a practitioner is required to perform each year in order to maintain practical competency, it is prudent to consider the stage of NIPE experience. For example, a practitioner who has just completed the prerequisite training will require regular participation in the NIPE if they are to embed and hone their skills to a higher level. This only comes with the experience and confidence that develops from regular participation. A practice arena that encourages such development not only assists confidence levels to rise, but also enables those areas of the NIPE, such as the hip examination, that need a high level of competency to be fine-tuned as the practitioner's expertise grows.

The onus is therefore not only on each individual practitioner to recognise their need for consolidation and knowledge, but also for their employers to support staff development and access to areas where skill levels can be further developed to meet and maintain best practice. In relation to NIPE and professional practice, all members of the multi-professional team must work together to achieve a high standard of practice, smooth routes of referral and parental as well as professional support (Nursing and Midwifery Council, 2015).

4 Safeguarding

Figure 4.1 Safeguarding assessment framework: the three domains of good assessment.
Source: UK Department of Education (2015a, p.22). This is reproduced with kind permission through Crown Copyright, 2010 from the Working Together to Safeguard Children publication. Contains public sector information licensed under the Open Government Licence v3.0.

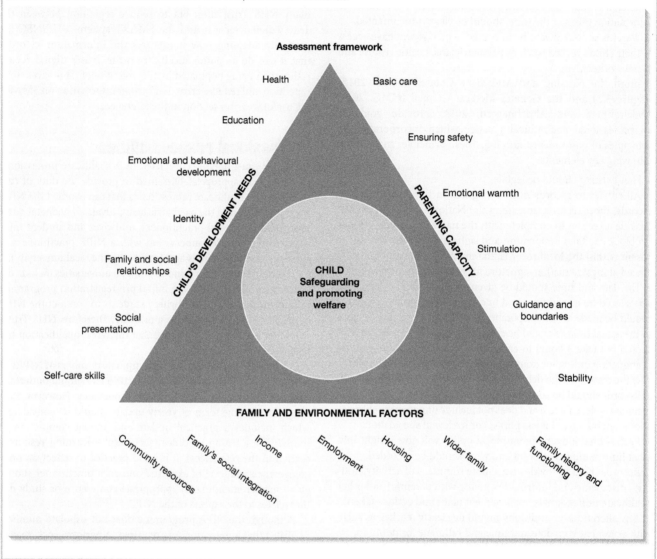

Safeguarding and promoting the welfare of children is defined as:

• Protecting children from maltreatment;
• Preventing impairment of children's health or development;
• Ensuring that children grow up in circumstances consistent with the provision of safe and effective care; and
• Taking action to enable all children have the best outcomes (UK Department for Education, 2015a, p.5).

Local Safeguarding Children Boards (LSCBs) were set up as a result of the Children Act 2004 and have the role of reviewing safeguarding procedures and the promotion of welfare from the perspectives of multi-agency and partnership working.

The practitioner performing the physical examination of the newborn has an important role in safeguarding. The potential for safeguarding problems is significant. In 2013–2014, over 650 000 children in England were referred to local authority children's social care services by individuals who had concerns about their welfare (UK Department for Education, 2015a, p.7). Additionally, under the provision of the Children Act 2004, any disabled child, refugee or asylum seeker automatically becomes a child in need (UK Department of Education, 2015a, p.18), to be referred to appropriate specialist support from the local authority.

The National Institute for Health and Care Excellence (NICE) (2012a) provide guidelines on factors that may contribute towards the vulnerability of children. NICE (2012a) also advises that care is taken to appreciate that circumstances vary and that not all children in vulnerable groups will be affected: and, neither will every vulnerable child fit neatly into any one category. Listed here are those factors that may be identified as relevant at the time of the physical examination:

• Parental drug and alcohol problems;
• Parental mental health problems;
• Family relationship problems, including domestic violence;
• Parental criminality;
• Single parent families;
• Parents aged under 18 years;
• Parents who have low educational attainment;
• Parents who are, or have ever been, in the care system;
• Children who have physical disabilities;
• Children likely to have speech, language and communication difficulties.

Protection from maltreatment and the provision of safe care may have necessitated assessment processes (Figure 4.1) beginning antenatally in order that the protection can begin from birth. The Childrens' Social Care (CSC) agencies will accept referrals from as early as a fetus reaching 18–20 weeks' gestation. As a result, the decision may already have been taken to place the newborn under local authority care through a Protection Order when the newborn examination is carried out. The plan of care may involve removal of the baby from the parents at birth or prior to leaving the maternity unit – either with parental consent or through a Court Order. This concerns newborns when evidence of vulnerability is significant enough that it is considered to be an immediate risk, such as:

• Known child protection concerns, possibly linked to a sibling;
• Current criminal status; and
• Health or disability concerns preventing parents from providing newborn care even within available support systems.

In some extreme cases of alcohol and/or substance abuse; physical or medical incapacity; learning disability; domestic violence; homelessness; or adverse social environments, it will be the rejection of support systems that may raise significant concerns for safeguarding.

Safeguarding is not only about those newborns already under local authority or social worker care. In most cases, the situation around vulnerability is more complex than an obvious requirement for a safety order. It will be important that support escalates appropriately through the referral to local authority agencies to enable effective local coordination and the assessment, intervention and/or targeted support as required (UK Department for Education, 2015b). On every occasion when an examination is carried out, the practitioner must follow local policy and protocols around how to access and check that neither the mother nor the infant has been named on any database or register associated with social care.

The role of the examiner is not only about safe care and protecting children from maltreatment, but there are also issues around preventing impairment of development, effective care and taking actions to enable best outcomes. All newborns must be considered from an individualised perspective with recognition that the examination itself could identify a disability, developmental or health concern. Prevention of potential impairment and optimising health and development from the examiners perspective, will be about ensuring that they can identify any potential risk to the infant. Plus, there will be the need to refer appropriately and initiate follow-up care alongside arranging further screening and diagnostics as required. Safeguarding includes the requirement to liaise and ensure that the infant has the best care and environment to fulfil his/her potential – both mentally and physically.

For the majority of newborns examined, achieving best outcomes and effective care will mostly involve the practitioner in providing highest standards of (evidence-based) health awareness: health education, instruction and advice for the parents/carers. Safeguarding will be about reinforcing government health agendas such as the use of car seats and immunisation programmes. It will be about encouraging best practice concerning infant feeding, bed sharing, smoking in the home, recognition of ill health and gaining early access to medical support. Health promotion is achieved when the parents embrace and comply with the advice given and the preventative measures encouraged – this must be individualised and relevant in order to optimise understanding and compliance. The links must be made between relevant history and risk factors. Understanding the risk factors will guide the individualisation of education and health promotion, with the aim of improving the family's ability to provide safe and effective care for their newborn.

5 Health promotion and education

Figure 5.1 Safe sleeping position.

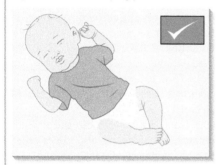
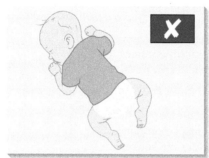
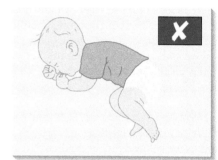

Figure 5.2 Feet to foot, not swaddled, arms free and no cot bumpers.

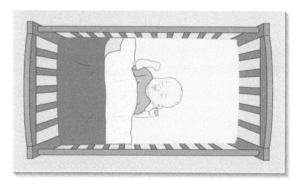

Table 5.1 Signs of neonatal cardiovascular and respiratory dysfunction.

Aspect	Signs
Respiration	Poor (gasping/irregular) or absent
Skin colour and mucous membranes	Pale or dusky (blue/grey) Mucous membranes of the mouth appear blue/very dark red
Tone	Floppy, inactive, poorly flexed
Attentiveness	Little recognition of surroundings, even though eyes are open, unresponsive

Any interaction between the practitioner and parents during daily care can provide an ideal opportunity to inform parents about their baby's health and development. This includes aspects such as normal neonatal reflexes, hearing and vision. However, the full physical examination of the newborn is a specific opportunity to inform parents about many *key* health promotion aspects: infant feeding; immunisation; signs of ill health (and actions to take); neonatal development; and support systems for parents. In addition, the evidence relating to best practice around specific topical issues can be promoted including use of car seats, passive smoking, reducing sudden infant death syndrome (SIDS) and positive parenting.

Feeding

Mode and frequency of feeding should be noted, including brand and amounts of any artificial formula. A normal 'output' (Box 5.1) will reinforce that the baby is obtaining adequate

Physical Examination of the Newborn at a Glance, First Edition. Denise (Dee) Campbell and Lyn Dolby.
© 2018 John Wiley & Sons, Ltd. Published 2018 by John Wiley & Sons, Ltd.

supplies of milk, particularly when breastfeeding. Assess whether normal frequency, colour and quantity of urine and meconium/stool have been noted.

Immunisation

Information should be shared regarding the UK Childhood Immunisation Programme. The practitioner should direct parents to the Personal Child Health Record ('Red') book as it contains information about the immunisation programme and the schedule for administration. However, parents should also be advised that they can gain further information from the Department of Health immunisation schedule website for details and updates (see useful website section in the references).

The bacille Calmette–Guérin (BCG) vaccination may be offered at birth if the newborn will travel to (or be visited by relatives from) an area with a high prevalence of tuberculosis. Maternity units will either offer this prior to discharge or refer parents to their GP for the vaccination (Box 5.2).

Sudden infant death syndrome

A total of 244 unexplained infant deaths (from birth to 12 months) occurred in England and Wales in 2011, of which almost two-thirds (64%) occurred in boys. Information sharing and the promotion of good practice in relation to 'safer sleeping' and 'tummy time' is essential in order to reduce the incidence of SIDS.

Supine position

Babies must always be placed on their backs to sleep. Reassure parents that there is no evidence that babies are at any greater risk of choking when lying in this position (Figure 5.1). However, 'tummy time' is still an important consideration and parents should be encouraged to allow their baby time (increasing with age) on his/her tummy. However, as soon as the parents leave the room or the baby falls asleep, he/she must be turned on to his/her back again.

Temperature

Room temperature should be 16–20°C. Overheating a newborn increases the risk of SIDS so babies must not be over-wrapped or at risk of being completely covered by bedding. They must not be swaddled, wear hats indoors, nor should duvets or cot bumpers be used. The baby should be placed with its feet touching the foot of the cot (Figure 5.2). The use of snowsuits should be restricted to outdoors and not used when in the car seat because of the inability to tighten the straps effectively.

Smoking

Thirty per cent of fetal deaths can be attributed to smoking in pregnancy. This risk is reduced if parents do not smoke in the same room as the baby, but it should be noted that some of the chemicals inhaled when smoking are exhaled over the following 2 hours.

Room sharing

The risk of SIDS is lower when the baby sleeps in a separate cot in the parental bedroom for the first 6 months of life.

Breastfeeding

Partial breastfeeding lowers the risk of SIDS but exclusive breastfeeding is associated with the lowest risk. Further information can be obtained from the Lullaby Trust (www.lullabytrust.org.uk).

Car seats and travel systems

The car seat should be used for the purpose intended – vehicle travel. The use of 'travel systems' enabling the car seat to be attached to a pram chassis should be restricted to periods of no longer than 1.5 hours. The car seat is purposely restrictive in order to reduce trauma in the event of an accident. It therefore reduces the movement of the baby, particularly of the hips, and prolonged restriction may affect hip development (see Chapter 44). Parents also need to be informed that it is crucial to consider where the seat belts on the baby car seat enter the back of the seat. When the baby is sitting in the seat, the insertion point of the belt in the back of the seat should be clearly visible, but as the baby grows this point of insertion will drop down out of view. This is the moment when the belt needs to be moved to the next insertion point, so that the possibility of trauma occurring during an accident is reduced.

Vitamin K administration

A deficiency of the vitamin K-dependent clotting factor can lead to spontaneous bleeding in the neonate, usually occurring near the end of the first week of life. Commonly, bleeding would be gastrointestinal and seen as haematemesis or melaena. It may also ooze from the umbilicus or become apparent because of a lack of clotting ability following trauma or circumcision. The routine administration of vitamin K to all babies has considerably reduced the incidence of haemorrhagic disease of the newborn.

Parents need to be supported to make an informed choice around intramuscular or oral administration – events during the antenatal–intrapartum period may make one route more advisable than the other (e.g. prolonged second stage of labour or traumatic delivery).

Signs of ill health

Babies contract harmless infections such as colds and sniffles which provide an important stimulus to their immune system. However, there are signs of ill health that are more serious and parents should be enabled to recognise these and act appropriately.

The key signs generally relate to poor cardiovascular or respiratory function and are highlighted in Table 5.1.

Parents must be reassured that significant ill health is rare but requires urgent response. They may be tired and have experienced major changes to their lives so may not remember every detail shared. However, studies have shown that when events occur, it is the parents that have been informed about what to watch out for who tend to respond quickest and most appropriately.

Next assessment

As part of the neonatal screening programme, all babies have a full physiological assessment performed within 72 hours of birth. A second assessment, at approximately 6–8 weeks of age, is performed by the GP. The latter examination aligns with the complete transition from fetus to neonate.

Promoting the health and well-being of the neonate is an important role and should not be underestimated. The information given will increase parental awareness of their child's abilities and future needs and may also reduce neonatal morbidity and mortality.

6 Communication during the examination

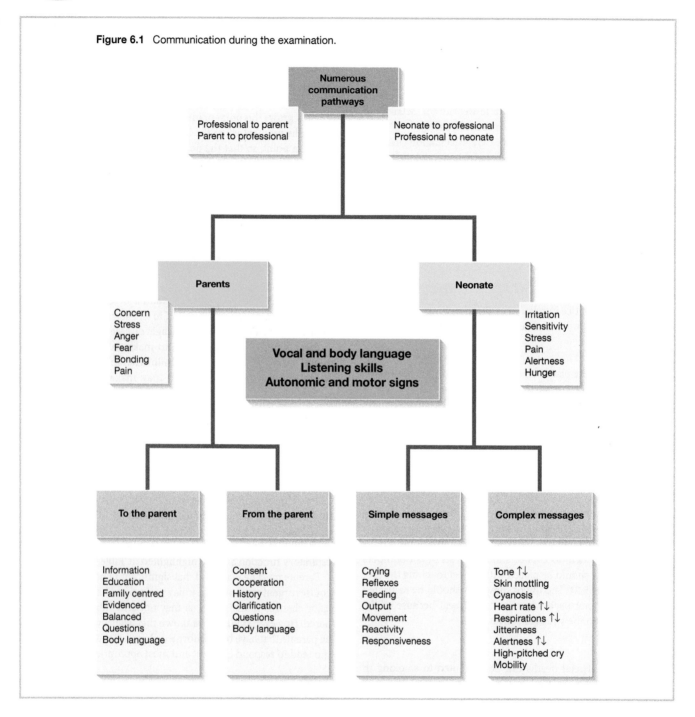

Figure 6.1 Communication during the examination.

Numerous communication pathways

Professional to parent
Parent to professional

Neonate to professional
Professional to neonate

Parents

Concern
Stress
Anger
Fear
Bonding
Pain

Neonate

Irritation
Sensitivity
Stress
Pain
Alertness
Hunger

**Vocal and body language
Listening skills
Autonomic and motor signs**

To the parent

Information
Education
Family centred
Evidenced
Balanced
Questions
Body language

From the parent

Consent
Cooperation
History
Clarification
Questions
Body language

Simple messages

Crying
Reflexes
Feeding
Output
Movement
Reactivity
Responsiveness

Complex messages

Tone ↑↓
Skin mottling
Cyanosis
Heart rate ↑↓
Respirations ↑↓
Jitteriness
Alertness ↑↓
High-pitched cry
Mobility

Physical Examination of the Newborn at a Glance, First Edition. Denise (Dee) Campbell and Lyn Dolby.
© 2018 John Wiley & Sons, Ltd. Published 2018 by John Wiley & Sons, Ltd.

There are numerous communication pathways that need to be considered during the examination. These are expanded upon in the text but an introductory overview can be seen in Figure 6.1.

Communicating with the neonate

Communication with the neonate may initially seem an unusual aspect to encourage. However, the practitioner is not seeking consent or attempting a verbal conversation. This is about 'hearing' the messages expressed through the body language, movements and noises made by the neonate. These will relate to levels of alertness, irritation, sensitivity, comfort, stress and even pain. They may relate to a psychological state or a physical condition and vary from a normal hunger cry to symptoms of an abnormality.

Every neonate is different and will demonstrate varying amounts of irritation, sensitivity and stress during the examination. Often, there will be obvious predisposing factors linked to the behaviour, such as the hungry baby who is difficult to console. However, the practitioner should always be alert to those communications that are less readily explained and indicate a need for further screening or diagnostic consideration. This could be a sound such as a hoarse, weak or high-pitched cry. It could be a physical sign of distress, linked to a particular movement or aspect of the examination. These should all inform the examination.

Irritation, sensitivity, stress and pain may be displayed through single aspects such as crying, or a more complex system of autonomic and motor signs that include skin mottling or reddening; increased respiration; jerky movements; arching or unusual stretching of limbs; high-pitched cries; jitteriness, startles or tremors. Similarly, immobility, flaccidity, uneven body tone or a lack of response to stimuli are also worrying 'messages' indicating a decreased level of alertness and responsiveness.

It is important that the practitioner understands the messages from the neonate and alters the management of the examination accordingly. In most cases this will not be an unhealthy baby but the examination itself that is causing irritation, over-stimulation or stress. Early awareness of the signs and a change in approach is both for the neonate's comfort and so that the examination can be completed.

This is also an opportunity to share information with the parents – to help them understand their baby's communications through observation of the individual behaviours. Simple things like moving the neonate from being under a direct light source; placing a warm hand gently on his/her head; covering the baby with clothing; applying or removing eye contact; gentle rocking or allowing a rest period; talking gently or keeping quiet can all be considered. Sometimes it is necessary to postpone the examination until after more immediate needs (such as feeding) have been satisfied.

Communicating with the parents

Analysis of the full history will inform the physical examination. This history will need to be confirmed, clarified and may be enlarged upon by the mother. The examination cannot be performed without her informed consent and cooperation throughout. The practitioner will need to apply family-centred communication, demonstrating full awareness of body language,

good listening skills and the ability to explain, detail and balance the information shared. These general principles should include ensuring the mother is comfortable and feels able to give her concentration to the conversation in an environment conducive to the sharing of information.

Informed consent

There are a number of essential elements to include when seeking consent for the physical examination. This begins with introductions and an explanation of the qualification to perform the examination. Opportunities must be given for the parents to raise concerns, ask questions and share further details. There should be awareness that the need for consent is ongoing throughout the examination. To enable 'informed' consent, the reasons for and benefits of the examination should be given but also with details on:

- Process – head to toe, opportunistic and health promotion.
- Timing – before 72 hours / 6–8 weeks; between feeds; time it takes.
- Components – where; what is examined; use of ophthalmoscope.
- Limitations of screening – false positives/negatives; aspects not included; ongoing neonatal development limiting results.
- Risks – possible stress; positive result; emergency management.
- Outcomes possible – apparently healthy; referral; further screening or diagnostic review; management of an identified condition.
- Further sources of information available.

Clarification and ongoing communications

The full review of the notes will have already taken place but, before the examination commences, this is an opportunity to check the accuracy of understanding, to ensure that nothing is missing or has changed from the records and to facilitate the parents sharing any concerns that they may have. The practitioner should use his/her skills of communication to appropriate questions and identify any evasive body language where supportive prompting may help. Specific questions should be asked to ascertain if any first degree relative or sibling has a history of any congenital abnormalities including heart or renal defects, developmental dysplasia of the hips or visual problems. There should be awareness of the sensitivity of any information shared.

Throughout the examination the communication should be a two-way conversation. Whilst it is important to take the opportunity to share information on health promotion and parenting skills, it should not become a 'lecture' from the practitioner (no matter how well-intentioned). Individualise the questions and information sharing; allow time for any reply – take the time to listen to what is said as well as observing body language cues.

It is important to appreciate that the parents are also listening intently to what the practitioner says and are also watching the practitioner's body language. Practitioners should beware of using unfamiliar words without explaining their meaning and ensure that they do not give cause for alarm where none exists; for example, explain that the practitioner always listens to the heart in various places for up to a minute. The practitioner should say that they are happy to explain everything to the parents and will not 'hide' any concerns from them. Findings should be explained in detail at the end of the examination.

Communicating concerns to parents

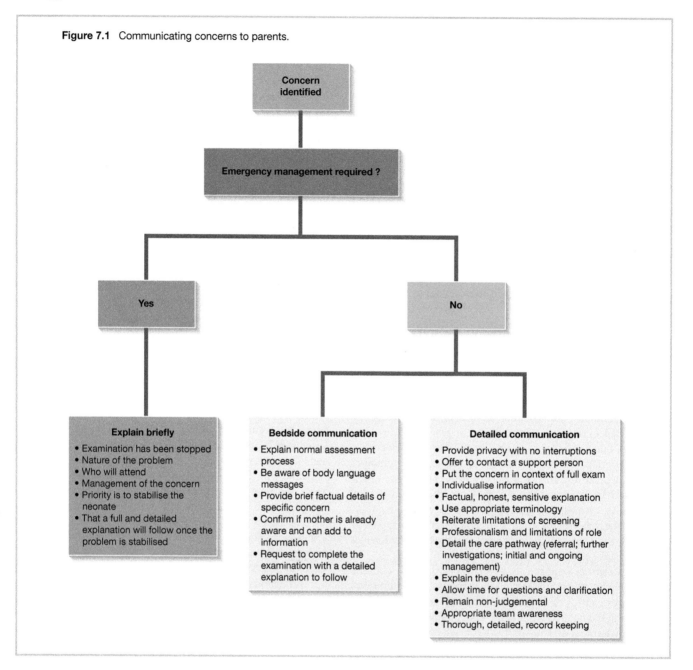

Figure 7.1 Communicating concerns to parents.

Concern identified

Emergency management required ?

Yes

No

Explain briefly
- Examination has been stopped
- Nature of the problem
- Who will attend
- Management of the concern
- Priority is to stabilise the neonate
- That a full and detailed explanation will follow once the problem is stabilised

Bedside communication
- Explain normal assessment process
- Be aware of body language messages
- Provide brief factual details of specific concern
- Confirm if mother is already aware and can add to information
- Request to complete the examination with a detailed explanation to follow

Detailed communication
- Provide privacy with no interruptions
- Offer to contact a support person
- Put the concern in context of full exam
- Individualise information
- Factual, honest, sensitive explanation
- Use appropriate terminology
- Reiterate limitations of screening
- Professionalism and limitations of role
- Detail the care pathway (referral; further investigations; initial and ongoing management)
- Explain the evidence base
- Allow time for questions and clarification
- Remain non-judgemental
- Appropriate team awareness
- Thorough, detailed, record keeping

Physical Examination of the Newborn at a Glance, First Edition. Denise (Dee) Campbell and Lyn Dolby.
© 2018 John Wiley & Sons, Ltd. Published 2018 by John Wiley & Sons, Ltd.

Communicating concerns to parents

Inevitably, there will be occasions when the examination identifies either a potential, or actual, physical abnormality or concern. If this is an emergency situation, then the examination is stopped and immediate management of the concern is required. However, in most situations, the examination can continue to allow all further information to be gleaned and included in the full analysis of the neonate's condition (Figure 7.1).

Be aware that even the most skilful practitioner will often give away clues of a problem to the parents through his/her body language, even when the smallest of concerns is identified. Whilst some information may need to be shared immediately, ideally the fully completed examination is required to determine the full extent of any problem and to ensure there are no other problems. The parents will be confused by a 'changing story' in which the problem described initially is found later to be less important. Nor will they maintain confidence in a practitioner when the scenario described is continually changing or worsening as the examination progresses.

It is also important that there is full appreciation of how the information about the concern is shared. This includes the terminology and intonation used, as well as the involvement of supportive body language. This balance of communications will ensure that it is not just 'what is said' but also 'how it is said' that will support the parents.

The practitioner should be prepared for questions and some anxiety from the parents. Questions should be answered factually and with honesty but taking care to avoid assumptions and generalisations. In most cases, it is advisable to explain the benefits of finishing the examination so that all the relevant factors can be screened for and a full understanding of the concern be known. This will prevent the sharing of misleading information with the parents and also reduces the risk of causing them undue worry. This will also give the mother some time to digest that there is a problem. Plus, it allows an opportunity to move to a more private area for the discussion where the likelihood of disturbance is minimised.

The practitioner should appreciate his/her limitations and not cross professional boundaries. He/she should be honest about the limits of his/her expertise and share with the parents any involvement to be expected from more senior or specialist practitioners. This may include lack of experience in breaking bad news – in which case arranging for a more experienced colleague to join in during the information sharing may be beneficial for the parents too. When appropriate, the practitioner should reiterate information around false positive results linked to the current concern and detail the care pathway that will now be followed. This should include specific information around any referral to be made (to whom, when and how), as well as any further screening or diagnostic investigations to be requested (by whom, when and what this will entail). If required, consider whether a senior paediatric referral can be expedited – this is often more feasible for the first examination and when the mother and baby are still within inpatient care.

The practitioner should be aware of the possible impact of any bad news and of approaches that can be used to reasonably limit distress. Time should be taken to seek assurances that the mother understands the degree of the problem but this must be with an awareness that every parent will react differently. Whilst the examination may have only revealed a medically insignificant problem, each parent brings to the discussion various factors that will influence their degree of reaction and this can be both positive and negative. For example, if antenatal screening has introduced the possibility of a severe abnormality being present, then news of a more minor one will be received positively. However, identifying the same minor concern where there was no prior awareness can be devastating for new parents. Additionally, the mother may have any number of aspects affecting both her ability to disseminate the information shared and how she responds. New parenthood is not always a time of joy – emotions can be affected by being postoperative, sleep deprived or in pain, let alone being negatively affected by transitional hormones or having socio-economic worries. Cultural, ethnic and social issues can also affect the initial responses and outward display of emotion. It is important that communication remains non-judgemental of any reaction displayed.

If there is any interim management or aspects of ongoing care that the neonate will benefit from, the parents need to be made aware of these and supported to be involved in providing this care. This could involve monitoring feeding (during periods of jaundice) or changes to nappy care routines when developmental dysplasia of the hip is suspected.

It may be appropriate for the practitioner to offer to contact the husband or partner or an alternative family member or friend if they are not with the mother at the time of the examination. The practitioner should then return when they have arrived to explain the findings of the examination and answer any further questions. Even when both parents are present initially, it is likely that after some time to accept that there is a problem, the family will appreciate further time for questions and discussion.

Coping with anger or aggression

In some rare cases, the reaction of one or more of the parents will involve anger or aggression. Dealing with bad news can be influenced by the physiological response of the body to the fears brought on by the bad news – a 'fight or flight' reaction. Additionally, attempts to cope may lead to self-preservation actions and wanting to apportion blame. This may also be about prior social learning and a lack of alternative coping strategies for the individual.

In the majority of cases, the aggression will not be physical and it will diffuse just as quickly as it occurred. Nonetheless, the practitioner should employ approaches to guarantee his/her safety which may be used to diffuse the situation. Initially, the practitioner may need to wait to allow the parents an opportunity to express their views. When responding, the practitioner should speak quietly in a calm voice, maintaining a non-threatening body posture with lowered eyes (directed at chin height) and relaxed arms. If there is any risk of physical aggression the practitioner should withdraw from the situation and employ team support for the situation, applying Trust policies for dealing with aggression.

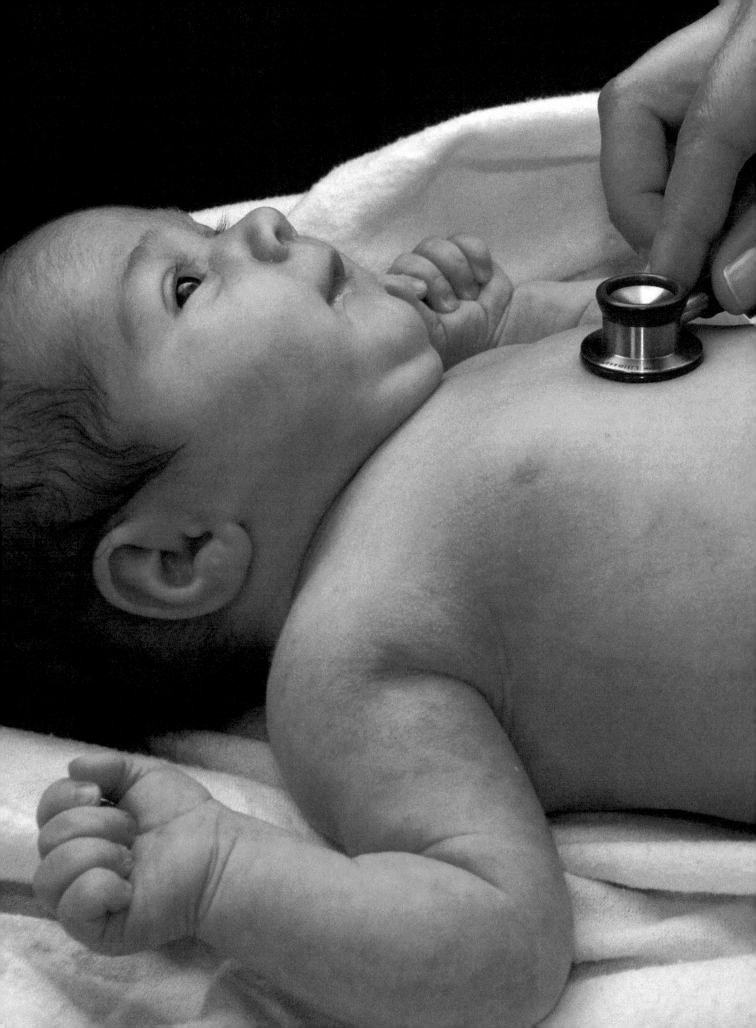

Neonatal physiology and pathophysiology

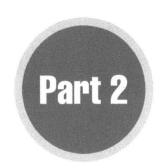

Part 2

8 Adaptation to neonatal life

Figure 8.1 The normal fetal and newborn heart.

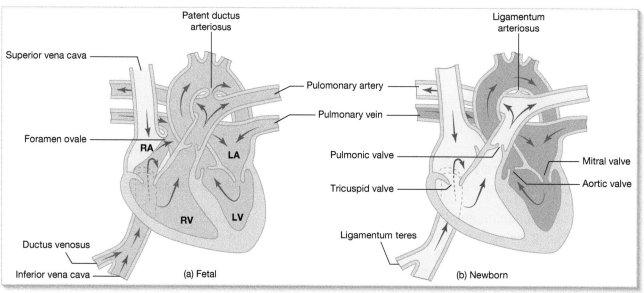

Table 8.1 The three key structures involved in fetal to neonatal adaptation.

Structure	Role
Ductus venosus	'Venosus' – a shunt connecting vein to vein Carries blood with a high oxygen content (80% O_2 saturation) from the placenta, through the fetal abdominal wall Shunts blood directly to the inferior vena cava Regulates blood flow via a sphincter Closes when blood flow in the umbilical vein reduces and stops When no longer in use, deposition of connective tissue within the duct lumen causes its closure and forms the ligamentum venosum
Foramen ovale	A flap (opening left to right) in the septum between the right and left atrium Shunts high O_2 concentration blood from areas of high pressure to low pressure Closes when pulmonary resistance decreases as blood is sent to the lungs; decreased pressure on right side of heart with a corresponding increased pressure on the left side of the heart Initial closure is caused by the pressure changes keeping the flap functionally closed until deposition of fibrous tissue creates a permanent closure, the fossa ovale
Ductus arteriosus	Shunts blood from pulmonary artery to aorta Protective function: • Damage to fetal lungs could occur in the event of circulatory overload • Enables strengthening of the right ventricle Carries medium O_2 saturated blood Development is influenced by maternal prostaglandin levels and resistance created by non-functioning lungs Closes when prostaglandin levels start to diminish, lungs expand and resistance is reduced, O_2 levels become elevated Bradykinin also assists in duct closure in the presence of high O_2 levels. It is released by lungs on inflation and acts to contract smooth muscle of the duct Constricts from birth, usually closes fully within the first 24–48 hours of life – results in ligamentum arteriosus

Table 8.2 Changes occurring from fetal to adult structures.

Fetal structure	Adult structure
Ductus venosus	Ligamentum venosum
Foramen ovale	Fossa ovalis
Ductus arteriosus	Ligamentum arteriosus
Umbilical vein	Ligamentum teres
Umbilical arteries and abdominal ligaments	Medial umbilical ligaments Superior vesicular artery (supplies the bladder)

Physical Examination of the Newborn at a Glance, First Edition. Denise (Dee) Campbell and Lyn Dolby.
© 2018 John Wiley & Sons, Ltd. Published 2018 by John Wiley & Sons, Ltd.

A complex chain of physiological events start to occur in the fetus in order to enable it to make the transition from intrauterine to extrauterine life. Most fetuses will make the journey into the outside world with little effect from the episodes of mild hypoxaemia that they may experience during labour. However, in the event of cardiorespiratory depression at birth, prompt recognition and effective resuscitation is paramount (see Chapter 10).

Fetal respiratory and cardiovascular development

Preparation for active use of the lungs occurs in the fetus from 10 weeks' gestation when breathing movements start to occur even though the lung tissue has minimal blood flow and the lungs are in a state of collapse. At approximately 24 weeks' gestation, the secretion of surfactant (a surface-active lipoprotein) commences and begins to coat the internal lining, reducing surface tension. The presence of surfactant enables easier initial lung expansion at birth and aids collapse and expansion as the lungs commence continuous use as an organ of gaseous exchange. Although in utero the lungs contain roughly 50 mL fluid, by birth this volume has already started to decrease and approximately 25% of this fluid will be expelled via the trachea during birth.

By 3 weeks' gestation, the fetal cardiovascular system has started to develop. In the absence of particular risk factors that may interfere with physiological progression (see Chapter 39), normal development continues throughout pregnancy.

In the fetus, the source of oxygen is the placenta which allows the blood arriving via the two umbilical arteries to become oxygenated. This oxygenated blood is then carried to the fetal heart by the umbilical vein where it is pumped round the fetus before eventually returning to the heart to be pumped once more to the placenta for oxygenation. The ductus arteriosus, foramen ovale and the ductus venosus act to reduce blood flow to the lungs whilst enabling the majority of oxygenated blood to pass to the major organs (Table 8.1). Only a small amount of oxygenated blood is required by the lungs to allow growth and development in readiness for extrauterine (adult) life (Table 8.2 and Figure 8.1).

Fetal to neonatal adaptation

Preparation for effective lung expansion is encouraged by to the creation of a negative intrathoracic pressure and an increased external atmospheric pressure alongside an accelerated production of surfactant in order to inhibit atelectasis. At birth, two-thirds of the lung liquid has already been expelled or is absorbed into the neonatal bloodstream or lymphatics within a few minutes of birth. The change in temperature (from the warm uterine environment to the cooler outside air) and the physical stimulus of light, touch and sound cause the central nervous system to react. Chemical stimulus in the form of dramatic increases in the levels of serum cortisol, antidiuretic hormone (ADH), thyroid-stimulating hormone (TSH) and catacholomines (neurotransmitters) serve to initiate breathing (Lissauer et al., 2014).

Occlusion of the umbilical cord effectively closes down the low pressure exerted by the placenta. With the first gasp, the lungs expand and pulmonary vascular resistance is further reduced as the pulmonary vessels dilate, increasing arterial oxygen tension. As a result, systemic vascular resistance increases and reducing blood flow to the ductus venosus causes it to constrict within minutes of birth. Deposition of connective tissue within the entire ductus lumen starts within days after birth with permanent structural closure usually being completed by 1–3 months of age.

The increased pulmonary circulation raises the pressure in the left atrium, forcing the septum primum against the septum secundum, thus causing the gradual closure of the foramen ovale. However, functional closure brought about by proliferation of fibrous tissue will not occur for some days, allowing some mixing of oxygenated and deoxygenated blood to occur. If the condition of coarctation of the aorta occurs (congenital heart condition), steroidal therapy to prevent functional closure of the foramen ovale and enable the continuation of the mixing of oxygenated and deoxygenated blood can buy some time for the neonate until surgical treatment can be performed.

The ductus arteriosus acts as a shunt from the descending aorta to the left pulmonary artery near the bifurcation of the pulmonary trunk. During fetal life, the low PaO_2 and the vasodilatory effect of circulating prostaglandins (PGE2) maintains the patency of the duct. However, after birth, when pulmonary oxygen saturation increases and circulatory PGE2 reduces, this shunt closes. In the term neonate, this closure usually occurs within the first 24–48 hours of life. Permanent closure occurs from fibrosis of the shunt, which takes 4–6 weeks to complete and this remnant of fetal life is then referred to as the ligamentum arteriosum.

Persistent pulmonary hypertension of the newborn

Persistent pulmonary hypertension of the newborn (PPHN), also known as persistent fetal circulation, is now relatively rare because of early recognition of those conditions that predispose to its appearance. PPHN occurs when either right-to-left ductal or atrial shunting persists after birth or when both occur in the presence of elevated right ventricular pressure.

Predisposing conditions include intrauterine hypoxia and ischaemia, respiratory distress syndrome, meconium aspiration syndrome, overwhelming sepsis and/or neonatal hypoxia and ischaemia. PPHN can cause severe hypoxaemia, which can result in increased levels of morbidity and mortality. However, better understanding and early recognition of the condition, improvements within antenatal and neonatal care, stringent monitoring of oxygen levels and blood pressure, plus prudent use of surfactant therapy has reduced the incidence of this potentially life-threatening condition.

Conditions that affect neonatal adaptation

The neonatal temperature is not stable at birth and the baby must metabolise (non-shivering thermogenesis) glucose stores in order to create heat. Therefore, if the baby cools, has reduced glucose stores or an infection, it is difficult to maintain minimal metabolic rate and oxygen needs (Waldron and Mackinnon, 2007).

Heat generated through non-shivering thermogenesis requires increased consumption of glucose and oxygen. If the baby continues to become chilled, his/her oxygen usage may exceed that of the levels available in air. As a result, metabolic acidosis can occur and the baby may show signs of cyanosis and tachypnoea. If the baby continues to be compromised and becomes hypoglycaemic, constriction of the pulmonary vessels and reduced surfactant levels can lead to respiratory distress. Neonatal physiology may try to address this situation by re-opening the foramen ovale, re-creating the right-to-left shunt and ensuing PPHN.

Therefore continuous assessment of fetal to neonatal adaptation is important to enable the early recognition of conditions or circumstances that may interfere with this process.

9 Thermoregulation

Table 9.1 Prevention of neonatal hypothermia.

	Causes of hypothermia	Actions that reduce heat loss
Baby emerges from a warm uterine environment (37°C) to cooler external environment (approx. 21°C)	Large body surface area to weight ratio, newborn skin has little subcutaneous fat and is wet at birth leading to immediate loss of heat to the environment	Turn off fans and keep doors closed to reduce the likelihood of draughts If appropriate, increase room temperature Dry the baby thoroughly with warm towels Dress in warm clothes or place skin to skin with mother Put a hat on the baby for at least 6 hours post birth
	Limited capacity to generate heat	A healthy term neonate should have enough brown adipose (fat) tissue to allow the process of 'non-shivering thermogenesis' to take place and thereby generate heat
		A newborn has an extremely limited or non-existent ability to shiver and therefore cannot use shivering to produce heat

Figure 9.1 Environmental heat loss.

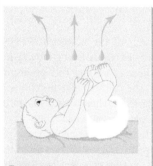

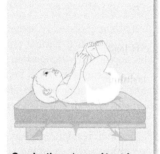

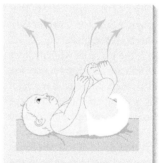

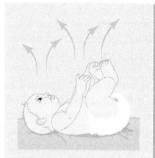

Evaporation – Loss of heat when liquid is converted to vapour (e.g. wet skin, wet nappy).

Conduction – Loss of heat from the body surface to cooler surface in direct contact (e.g. cold towels; mattress; weighing scales).

Convection – Loss of heat from body surface to cooler air (draughts through open windows, doors and fans).

Radiation – Loss of heat from the body surface to a cooler solid surface that is not in direct contact, but in close proximity to the body (cold objects near to baby; e.g. cot sides).

Figure 9.2 The energy triangle.

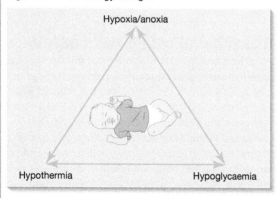

Hypoxia/anoxia

Hypothermia

Hypoglycaemia

Physical Examination of the Newborn at a Glance, First Edition. Denise (Dee) Campbell and Lyn Dolby.
© 2018 John Wiley & Sons, Ltd. Published 2018 by John Wiley & Sons, Ltd.

Normal core body temperature is usually classified as 36.5–37.4°C, whereas a temperature of 34–36.4°C is viewed as mild hypothermia and 32–35.9°C as severe hypothermia (Sinha *et al.*, 2012).

Measuring the skin temperature will give a lower reading to that of 'core' temperature. Using a digital thermometer, if used and calibrated correctly, can give a more accurate recording than a disposable thermometer. However, a non-touch infrared temperature measurement may be found to be an accurate and cost-effective method in the future (Sollai *et al.*, 2016).

A healthy term neonate should be able to regulate his/her temperature soon after birth. Initially, a natural increase in metabolic rate will assist in maintaining a normal core body temperature but the duration of this status is dependent on a number of environmental factors. A drop of 1–2°C per minute (Sinha *et al.*, 2012) can occur during the immediate post birth period in the event of intrapartum compromise or when steps are not taken to protect the neonate from the colder extrauterine environment. A baby who becomes hypothermic may take 4–8 hours to regain a normal body temperature (Black and Rose, 2000). Significant hypothermia in preterm babies increases mortality by 60%. However, a baby who has been compromised during labour, whose weight is less than expected for gestational age or who has an underlying sepsis or be suffering from shock may not have the quantity of, or the ability to metabolise, its store of brown adipose tissue and as a consequence is more at risk of hypothermia.

Mechanism of heat loss

In utero, the fetus has no need for thermoregulation within the warm confines of the womb (usually a constant 0–5°C above maternal temperature). However, at birth, the immaturity of the thermoregulatory system does not allow for adult reactions to cold such as shivering. Therefore action taken at birth can help maintain a normal core body temperature by preventing heat loss from occurring as a result of evaporation, conduction, convection and radiation (Figure 9.1). Quick assessment of the birthing room environment as the second stage of labour approaches should indicate if the room is warm enough, if windows need closing or a fan needs to be turned off.

Neonatal response to cold stress

When a baby is exposed to a cold environment a series of physiological responses occur in order to aid the conservation of body heat:

- **Peripheral vasoconstriction** – reduces heat lost via the extremities by decreasing the amount of blood within the circulatory system passing through the extremities.
- **Increased heat production** – through increased metabolic rate occurs but this also necessitates a rise in oxygen consumption and if the fetus developed hypoxia in utero this may reduce the efficiency of this action.
- **Increased voluntary and involuntary muscular activity – shivering** – in preterm infants shivering is virtually non-existent and in term infants the ability to shiver is limited. Hypoxia and resultant acidosis in utero will impact on this ability and when glucose levels may not be in plentiful supply, because of the natural initial reduction in levels soon after birth or an inborn error of metabolism, lead to further adverse impacts.
- **Non-shivering thermogenesis** – during the last trimester of pregnancy, brown adipose tissue (BAT) is deposited primarily around the neck, axilla, scapulae, sternum, adrenals and the kidneys of the fetus. BAT is a highly specialised type of adipose tissue that is well vascularised and the cells are densely packed with mitochondria, which are the power houses behind cellular activity.

Hypothermia (neonatal cold injury)

Hypothermia is one of the three major considerations within the 'energy triangle' (Figure 9.2). The close relationship between hypothermia, hypoglycaemia and hypoxia/anoxia must never be underestimated and understanding the interactions between these three factors and the impact on the newborn baby is paramount. The midwife needs to recognise when intrapartum compromise has occurred and be vigilant in assessing and facilitating the baby's adaptation to extrauterine life and thermal regulation (for more detailed information on the energy triangle see Aylott 2006).

Both oxygen consumption and utilisation of glucose will be increased in the event of prolonged exposure to cold and this leads to increasing levels of hypoxia and hypoglycaemia. Peripheral cyanosis will occur in an attempt to maintain core body temperature. Initially, the neonate may have been vocally signalling his/her discomfort, but as the baby becomes colder lethargy and an unwillingness to feed will soon become evident.

If the condition continues unrecognised, the neonate may develop apnoeic spells which further reduce oxygen levels and exacerbate respiratory distress syndrome. On re-warming, the baby's physiological response to the improvement in blood pressure and perfusion is to wash out the products of anaerobic metabolism into the circulation, thereby causing metabolic acidosis. Hypoglycaemia occurs because of the increased demand for glucose in a baby whose reserves may already be running low. Therefore, in severe cases or in babies who weigh less than expected for their gestational age (who may have less BAT), regular blood glucose monitoring and appropriate management is essential to maintain adequate levels of circulating glucose.

Actions to prevent hypothermia

Prevention of hypothermia is relatively easy in the healthy term neonate. The actions that can be taken to reduce the risk of hypothermia are as stated by Waldron and Mackinnon (2007), often iatrogenic, and are summarised in Table 9.1. Drying the baby thoroughly, use of a hat (as hair may still be slightly damp) and placing the baby skin to skin with one of the parents after birth is highly recommended as best practice. Not only do such actions promote the stabilisation of the baby's temperature by reducing radiant and conductive heat loss, but it also encourages bonding and breastfeeding.

If a baby has been warmed after becoming mildly hypothermic, his/her ability to maintain temperature needs to be tested before being discharged home. An inability to maintain a normal core body temperature can indicate an underlying morbidity. It should also be noted that a baby may exhibit cutis marmorata (a mottling of the skin, often in the lower extremities) which is a vascular response in a baby who is re-warming after having been cold for a period of time. However, if this condition persists, further investigation is required as it may indicate poor perfusion as the result of developing sepsis, or it can be associated with trisomy 21, Edwards' (trisomy 18) and Cornelia de Lange syndromes.

10 Resuscitation of the newborn

Figure 10.1 Algorithm for newborn life support.
Source: Reproduced with the kind permission of the Resuscitation Council (UK), 2015.

Resuscitation Council (UK) | GUIDELINES 2015 | Newborn Life Support

Maintain temperature

(Antenatal counselling)
Team briefing and
equipment check

↓

Birth

↓

Dry the baby
Maintain normal temperature
Start the clock or note the time

↓

Assess (tone), **breathing,
heart rate**

↓

If gasping or not breathing:
Open the airway
Give 5 inflation breaths
Consider SpO_2 ± ECG monitoring

↓

Re-assess
If no increase in heart rate look for
chest movement during inflation

↓

If chest not moving:
Recheck head position
Consider 2-person airway control
and other airway manoeuvres
Repeat inflation breaths
SpO_2 ± ECG monitoring
Look for a response

Acceptable pre-ductal SpO_2	
2 min	60%
3 min	70%
4 min	80%
5 min	85%
10 min	90%

↓

If no increase in heart rate look
for chest movement

↓

When the chest is moving:
If heart rate is not detectable or
very slow (< 60 min^{-1}) ventilate
for 30 seconds

↓

Reassess heart rate
If still < 60 min^{-1} start chest
compressions; coordinate with
ventilation breaths (ratio 3:1)

↓

Re-assess heart rate
every 30 seconds
If heart rate is not detectable or
very slow (< 60 min^{-1}) consider
venous access and drugs

↓

Update parents and
debrief team

60 s

Increase oxygen (guided by oximetry if available)

AT
ALL
TIMES
ASK:
DO
YOU
NEED
HELP?

Figure 10.2 The neutral head position – essential for neonatal resuscitation.
Source: Lissauer and Fanaroff (2011). Reproduced with permission of John Wiley & Sons.

(a) ✓ (b) ✗ (c) ✗

Figure 10.3 Size and position of face masks.
Source: Lissauer and Fanaroff (2011). Reproduced with permission of John Wiley & Sons.

Correct ✓
Covers mouth, nose
and chin but not eyes

Incorrect ✗
Too large: covers eyes
and extends over chin

Incorrect ✗
Too small: does not
cover nose and
mouth completely

Figure 10.4 Sites for chest compression.
Source: Lissauer and Fanaroff (2011). Reproduced with permission of John Wiley & Sons.

Sternum
Nipple line
Compression area
Xiphoid

(a) Landmarks for chest compression

(b) Thumb technique for larger neonates: side by side

(c) Thumb technique for small neonates: one above the other

Sternum
Xyphoid
Nipple line

(d) Two finger technique

Resuscitation (UK Resuscitation Council, 2015)

This book relates to the postnatal period and physical examination of the newborn. However, with awareness that the early examinations commonly take place in birthing environments and that the practitioner could be called to assist at an emergency, the full approach to resuscitation is covered here.

Predisposing factors

Antenatal

- Acute hypoxic incident (e.g. abruptio placentae, eclampsia, maternal collapse, cord prolapse).
- Chronic hypoxia (e.g. pre-eclampsia, placental insufficiency, twin–twin transfusion).

Intrapartum

- Acute hypoxic incident (e.g. shoulder dystocia, intracranial haemorrhage, head entrapment, uterine rupture).
- Chronic hypoxic (e.g. cephalopelvic disproportion, prolonged labour).

Postnatal

- Acute hypoxic incident (e.g. accidental smothering, airway obstruction, vasovagal attack [poor suctioning], unclamped cord).
- Chronic hypoxia (e.g. hypothermia, pneumothorax, sepsis, abnormality [pressure or obstruction], hypoglycaemia, metabolic disorder, heart disease).

Physiology

It is rare for the neonate to have a cardiac arrest but this is possible when associated with heart disease or congenital cardiac malformation. On almost all occasions there will be primary respiratory arrest linked to hypoxia. The initial adaptive response of the respiratory centre to hypoxia will be to increase respiratory effort to compensate. If there is no response, *primary apnoea* will occur. Primitive respiratory centres in the spinal cord then stimulate *agonal gasping* efforts and the body shudders in a final attempt to inflate the lungs. If this fails, *terminal apnoea* will follow. The increasing levels of lactic acid also affect cardiac function and any bradycardia worsens until the heart stops.

Management (Figure 10.1)

Whenever possible, the area for resuscitation should be prepared in advance, equipment checked, the parents made aware (and consenting) and a paediatric team made available for support. The risk factors should be known (see Chapter 25), with particular attention to gestation, fetal compromise, abnormalities, maternal medication and meconium liquor. Throughout management it is essential to carry out the following.

- Note times (start the clock at birth).
- Assess breathing, heart rate (HR) and tone every 30 s.
- Keep the newborn warm and dry – hypothermia increases the likelihood of hypoglycaemia and acidosis. At birth, dry the newborn with a warm towel; replace the wet towel with a second dry one – this will also provide stimulation. Maintain temperature at 36.5–37.5°C using a hat to assist temperature control.
- Position appropriately – head in a neutral position (Figure 10.2) and chest clear to allow visualisation of response to resuscitation. A resuscitaire can provide the optimum environment including a clock, oxygen, suction, heat and pulse oximeter.

Airway management – newborn not breathing

- Head in *neutral position* – may require a towel beneath the shoulders, chin support, jaw thrust or airway.
- Check *airway patency* – suction is not required unless meconium, vernix caseosa or blood is directly visualised obstructing the airway.
- Apply correct-sized *mask* (Figure 10.3).
- Give *five inflation breaths* – using bag, valve, mask system connected to air supply (mix with oxygen if SpO_2 levels require it). Inflation pressure of 30 cm water for 2–3 s. Observe for chest movement – if not seen, reassess and follow guidelines for absence of chest expansion below. Then repeat *inflation breaths*.
- Progress to *ventilation breaths* at a rate of 30–40/min (once chest expansion has been seen at least 3 out of 5 inflation breaths).
- Even if HR not detectable or <60/min, give 30 s of ventilation before starting cardiac compressions as below.
- *Stop* ventilation when HR >100/min and breathing spontaneously.
- Monitor throughout with *pulse oximeter* on the right side – see Figure 10.1 for acceptable HR and SpO_2 levels.

Airway manoeuvres for absence of chest expansion

- Recheck head is in a neutral position.
- Chin support – to prevent head flexion.
- Jaw thrust – if newborn tone is poor.
- Two-person airway control – one holding the head, applying jaw thrust and holding the mask; the second operating the T-piece or bag.
- Guedel airway – to prevent tongue or soft tissue obstruction.
- Suction – laryngoscope (direct vision), paediatric Yankauer sucker.
- Intubation required if all other manoevres have failed.

Cardiac compressions – if HR <60 beats/min after 30 s of ventilation

- Must be effective ventilation for cardiac compression to work.
- *Encircle the chest* with two hands.
- Apply *pressure* with overlapping thumbs, to the lower third of the sternum, avoiding the ziphoid process (Figure 10.4).
- *Depress* by one-third of the chest's AP diameter.
- Allow full *expansion* of the chest between compressions so the heart refills.
- Rate is *3 : 1 cardiac compressions to ventilation breaths*; therefore 30 breathes and 90 compressions per minute.
- Use an ECG to continuously record HR (when available).
- *Stop* compressions when HR >60/minute.
- Consider *venous access and drugs* if HR <60 minute or not improving.

Drugs (S A D)

Drugs are used if no response is seen despite effective ventilation and cardiac compressions.

- Sodium bicarbonate – 4.2% solution; dose 1–2 mmol/kg IV.
- Adrenaline (epinephrine) 1 : 10 000 solution; dose 0.1–0.3 mL/kg IV or 0.3–1 mL/kg via endotracheal tube.
- Dextrose 10%; dose 2.5 mL/kg IV.
- Volume expander (if needed) – sodium chloride 0.9%; bolus dose of 10 mL/kg IV given over 10–20 s.

Stopping resuscitation

- Ideally, when HR >100 and spontaneous breathing is present.
- HR is not present or no longer present after 10 minutes of active resuscitation.

11 Hypoglycaemia

Figure 11.1 Glucose metabolism.

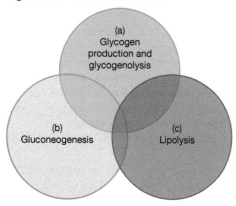

(a) Occurs mainly in the liver and muscles, but liver glycogen must be available (in fetus excess maternal glucose supplies are stored as glycogen in the liver)

(b) Substrates required here are amino acids (particularly) alanine, lactate, pyruvate and glycerol

(c) Glycerol is metabolised from adipose tissue to be directly used in gluconeogenesis in the neonate. Lipolysis releases fatty acids and triglycerides which are metabolised to ketone bodies   used directly in energy production   brain. Infant feeding (particularly breast milk) stimulates ketone body production

Table 11.1 Causes of hypoglycaemia.

Decreased levels of substrate	Premature babies Multiple births
Increased glucose requirements	Hyperinsulinaemia Baby of a diabetic mother Rhesus isoimmunisation Hypertropyhy of the pancreas (nesidioblastosis) Islet cell tumour Beckwith—Wiedemann syndrome Polycythaemia
Inability to utilise glucose	Glycogen storage disease Galactosaemia Fructose intolerance Inborn errors of meatabolism
Miscellaneous and/or accessory to	Birth asphyxia Endocrine deficiencies (e.g. congenial adrenal hyperplasia) Hypopituitarism

Table 11.2 At risk factors instigating immediate investigation and management.

Babies with a history of predisposing factors	Babies with one or more of the following conditions of the following clinical signs
Babies of diabetic mothers	Perinatal acidosis (cord arterial or infant pH <7.1 and base deficit >8 mmol [moderate] and >12 mmol [severe] metabolic acidosis)
	Hypothermia (<36.5°C)
Babies whose mothers have taken beta-blockers	Suspected or confirmed early onset sepsis
	Cyanosis
	Apnoea
	Seizures
Babies with intrauterine growth restriction (IUGR) with a birth weight ≤2nd centile BAPM includes term babies who have a 'clinically wasted' appearance as well as infants who are premature or part of a multiple birth	Hypotonia
	Lethargy
	Altered level of consciousness
N.B. The perameters **must** be measured using a gender-specific centile chart	High-pitched cry

A transient rise in fetal glucose concentrations from glycogenolysis and gluconeogenesis occurs close to the baby's birth. When birth occurs and the placental connection is lost, a rapid decline in neonatal glucose levels then follows, reaching a nadir at 1–2 hours of age. Without the steady maternal supply of glucose via the placenta, a strong ketogenic response is instigated through the processes involved in glucose metabolism (Figure 11.1). As a result, the blood glucose concentration rises again to a level similar to that in late fetal gestation at approximately 2–4 hours post birth. By 3–4 days post birth, the blood glucose level will have reached adult level. However, if any part of the process of glucose metabolism is disrupted, hypoglycaemia can rapidly develop (see Table 11.1 for causes of neonatal hypoglycaemia).

Hypoglycaemia occurs when the blood sugar concentration drops below a predetermined level, causing the appearance of clinical symptoms. It occurs in about 1–3 out of every 1000 births. However, there has been much discussion relating to how low the level of blood glucose can fall in relation to the baby's age before physiological compromise occurs, and research has been commissioned to explore the key factors that aid early recognition of the condition. For example, blood glucose levels ranging from 2.0 to 2.5 mmol/L have been quoted as acceptable (Sinha *et al.*, 2012; Hawdon, 2015). Therefore, it is important for practitioners to understand their own local guidelines in conjunction with understanding the baby's physiological responses to being detached from the placenta and becoming independent.

Most babies do not develop clinically significant hypoglycaemia as this condition occurs in babies who have impaired metabolic adaptation or as a result of increased demands for glucose in a baby whose reserves may already be running low. Therefore, in severe cases or in babies who weigh less than expected for their gestational age, regular blood glucose monitoring and appropriate management is essential in order to maintain adequate levels of circulating glucose.

Glucose and oxygen are the main sources of fuel utilised by the human brain. Without adequate blood sugar levels (or oxygen), the brain's ability to function is initially impaired. As the state of hypoglycaemia continues or becomes severe, there is an ever-increasing likelihood of seizures, permanent injury to the brain and long-term neurodevelopmental impairment. The necessity of appreciating the risk factors relating to hypoglycaemia and recognising the signs and symptoms relating to the condition is paramount. Indeed, Hawdon *et al.* (2017) discussed the rare cases of litigation that arose from a lack of early recognition or robust treatment protocols. This particular study was commissioned on behalf of the NHS Improvement Patient Safety Programme 'Avoiding harm leading to Term Admissions Into Neonatal units' (Atain). More recently, the NHS England Neonatal Hypoglycaemia Working Group in contribution with the NHS Improvement Patient Safety Programme commissioned an expert group to develop a national Framework for Practice. The first draft guidance was released for consultation in December 2016 (British Association for Perinatal Medicine; BAPM). This document seeks to provide more robust guidance relating to the recognition and treatment protocols for neonatal hypoglycaemia and should be embedded in the local protocols to be followed by all healthcare workers.

Predisposing factors

Immediate investigation and management should be instigated in babies who have known predisposing risk factors and/or in those who demonstrate one or more clinical signs (Table 11.2). However, 'jitteriness' is common in neonates and is not in itself an indication to measure blood glucose (jitteriness is witnessed as excessive repetitive movements of one or more limbs that are unprovoked and not in response to a stimulus). It should also be remembered that neonates do not display the usual autonomic nervous system response seen in adults, for example, sweating and pallor.

The working group (BAPM, 2017) also considered babies that are large for their gestational age. Their conclusion was that if there was no evidence of maternal diabetes and the baby did not have any of the dysmorphic features associated with Beckwith–Wiedemann syndrome, then routine screening for hypoglycaemia was not required. However, as with any baby, hypoglycaemia can be asymptomatic in its presentation. An apparently 'normal' baby may have a latent condition – such as infection – that may influence his/her requirement for energy and affect levels of circulating glucose. Therefore, any increase or decrease in temperature or abnormal feeding behaviour (e.g. not suckling effectively or waking for feeds, unsettled or demanding frequent feeds) that appears after a period of feeding well should prompt further assessment and investigation of blood glucose levels.

BAPM (2017) reiterate the importance that all babies should be assessed at birth for risk of hypoglycaemia. For those with risk factors, the BAPM Newborn Early Warning Trigger and Track (NEWTT) chart should be commenced as it gives a visual assessment of the baby's condition and is a useful aide in the detection of the hypoglycaemia. The NEWTT chart can be accessed on the BAPM publications website (https://www.bapm.org/sites/default/files/files/Front%20of%20chart%20final%20June15.pdf).

Blood glucose measuring equipment for the newborn

Diagnosis and treatment of neonatal hypoglycaemia requires the accurate measurement of blood glucose levels. Currently, significant inaccuracy can occur with current cot-side technology, particularly within the range 0–2.0 mmol/L. In the event that a handheld glucometer has to be used for blood glucose measurement, only devices that conform to ISO 15197:2013 and have been validated for neonatal use should be employed. However, even with such equipment there is a possible error of ±0.5 mmol/L for values <5.5 mmol/L.

The limitations of glucose meters can also become evident in the event of recording inaccurately high glucose results with low packed cell volume (PCV) samples or, conversely, low glucose results when the PCV is high. This is because of the movement and activity that occurs when glucose is diffused in water, resulting in whole blood glucose demonstrating a 10–15% lower level than with plasma glucose (depending on the haematocrit level). Consequently, measuring whole blood glucose values is advocated, particularly in the event of a low result being obtained, if the correct management is to be commenced. As a more accurate method of blood sugar measurement should be used, it is preferable for a ward-based blood gas biosensor to be available. Such equipment is not only considered the reference standard for accuracy in measuring whole blood glucose, but can also do so in a speedy and efficient manner.

Training and baby-friendly initiative

Hawdon *et al.* (2017) highlighted the need for the provision of adequate training for all those involved in neonatal care and new guidance to this effect was published by BAPM (2017). Such training should embrace the need to avoid separating mothers and babies and ultimately reduce unnecessary investigations in those babies not at risk and who do not demonstrate clinical signs. BAPM also advocate maternity units to adopt the UNICEF UK Baby Friendly standards tool (http://www.unicef.org.uk/babyfriendly/) to assist in training and assessment of feeding during the first week of life. The tool should help focus the attention of healthcare workers on the ability of the baby to feed, promote breastfeeding support and enable recognition of poor feeding that may contribute to hypoglycaemia.

12 Physiological jaundice

Figure 12.1 The process of bilirubin metabolism.

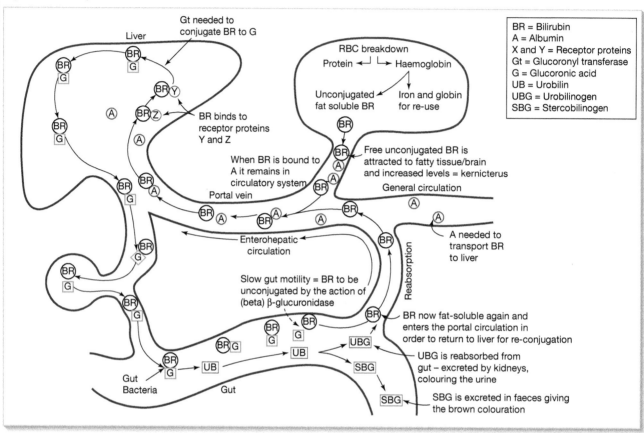

BR = Bilirubin
A = Albumin
X and Y = Receptor proteins
Gt = Glucoronyl transferase
G = Glucoronic acid
UB = Urobilin
UBG = Urobilinogen
SBG = Stercobilinogen

Gt needed to conjugate BR to G

Liver

RBC breakdown

Protein ← ⊣ → Haemoglobin

Unconjugated fat soluble BR   Iron and globin for re-use

BR binds to receptor proteins Y and Z

When BR is bound to A it remains in circulatory system

Free unconjugated BR is attracted to fatty tissue/brain and increased levels = kernicterus

Portal vein

General circulation

A needed to transport BR to liver

Enterohepatic circulation

Slow gut motility = BR to be unconjugated by the action of (beta) β-glucuronidase

Reabsorption

BR now fat-soluble again and enters the portal circulation in order to return to liver for re-conjugation

UBG is reabsorbed from gut – excreted by kidneys, colouring the urine

Gut Bacteria   Gut

SBG is excreted in faeces giving the brown colouration

Table 12.1 Factors that adversely affect bilirubin metabolism.

Site	Effect on bilirubin metabolism
Spleen	Increased haemolysis leads to excessive bilirubin levels
General circulation/portal vein	Shortage of plasma albumin to bind with unconjugated fat soluble bilirubin allows it to exit the circulatory system where, because of its attraction to fatty tissue/brain, high levels can cause kernicterus
Liver	Hypoxia and hypoglycaemia reduce the level of metabolism as both O_2 and glucose are necessary for the process to work. Glucose is the raw material used for the production of gluconoric acid
Liver → gall bladder	Biliary obstruction leads to obstructive jaundice Low levels of enteric bacteria
Gut	Slow gut mobility leads to bilirubin becoming unconjugated again because of the action of β-glucuronidase

Table 12.2 Management of physiological jaundice.

Positive actions	Negative symptoms
Skin to skin and early frequent feeds Observe quality of feed and willingness of baby to suckle and state of alertness/general well-being Frequent feeds even if baby needs to be woken for feeds (e.g. 3 hourly) Give expressed breast milk if necessary Supplementation with artificial formula milk – only if baby is unable to suckle	Depth of colour (yellow) is becoming more marked/widespread Baby is lethargic, sleepy, difficult to rouse Passage of 'pale' stools Baby demonstrates decreased muscle tone, high-pitched cry or increasing development of 'unusual' movement
N.B. Placing baby in sunlight (even indirectly/filtered) can cause dehydration from overheating and sunburn as the skin layer is thinner than that of an adult (Harrison *et al.*, 2005).	

Physical Examination of the Newborn at a Glance, First Edition. Denise (Dee) Campbell and Lyn Dolby.
© 2018 John Wiley & Sons, Ltd. Published 2018 by John Wiley & Sons, Ltd.

Physiological bilirubin metabolism

Physiological jaundice is the deposition of bilirubin (a weak, fat-soluble, yellow pigmented acid) in the newborn skin, sclera and mucous membranes (Stables and Rankin, 2010). Bilirubin is the by-product of bilirubin metabolism that marks the end of the lifespan of a red blood cell (RBC). This process of RBC destruction occurs in the reticuloendothelial system (liver, spleen and macrophages). When the level of serum bilirubin exceeds 90 µm/L, the characteristic yellow discoloration of the skin becomes visible (Sinha *et al.*, 2012) and may be a result of physiological, pathological conditions or breastmilk jaundice.

This chapter focuses on the physiological process of neonatal bilirubin metabolism. Entry of unconjugated bilirubin into the brain (causing the characteristic yellow staining of the tissue) can cause both short and long-term neurological dysfunction (bilirubin encephalopathy). The clinical features associated with acute or chronic bilirubin encephalopathy are collectively termed kernicterus. The risk of kernicterus increases in babies with extremely high bilirubin levels. Kernicterus is also known to occur at lower levels of bilirubin in term babies who have risk factors, and in preterm babies.

Incidence and risk factors

Babies who are more at risk of jaundice include those whose sibling was also jaundiced as a baby. Ethnicity is also a factor, depending on place of birth, as those with ethnic routes from Asia or South America (excluding those not born in their home country) would appear to have a greater propensity towards jaundice than those with European and African ancestry. In the UK, physiological jaundice occurs in approximately 50% of term babies each year. A much higher proportion of preterm babies (80%) will become jaundiced as a result of organ immaturity and accompanying disorders of prematurity.

During fetal life, the placenta and maternal liver manage fetal RBC breakdown. Although the fetus can conjugate small quantities of bilirubin, the fetal liver is relatively inactive, only taking over bilirubin metabolism at birth. The enzyme β-glucuronidase, present in the fetus' small-bowel luminal brush border, is released into the intestinal lumen, where it deconjugates bilirubin glucuronide. Free (unconjugated) bilirubin is then reabsorbed from the gastrointestinal tract and re-enters the fetal circulation. Fetal bilirubin is cleared from the circulation by placental transfer into the mother's plasma following a concentration gradient. The maternal liver then takes on the process of bilirubin metabolism by conjugating and excreting the fetal bilirubin until this placental connection is terminated at birth.

The neonatal liver continues to conjugate and excrete bilirubin into bile so it can be eliminated in the stool. However, because of the lack of intestinal bacteria for oxidising bilirubin to urobilinogen in the gut, the unaltered bilirubin remains in the stool, giving the typical bright yellow colour. In addition, the neonatal gastrointestinal tract (like that of the fetus) contains β-glucuronidase, which deconjugates some of the bilirubin. When the neonate is fed, the gastro colic reflex is stimulated, causing bilirubin to be excreted via the stools before most of it can be deconjugated and reabsorbed. Nevertheless, in many neonates, the unconjugated bilirubin is re-absorbed and returned to the circulation from the intestinal lumen (enterohepatic circulation of bilirubin), contributing to physiological hyperbilirubinaemia and jaundice.

Bilirubin metabolism

The process of bilirubin metabolism is shown in Figure 12.1, demonstrating the factors on which the process is dependent to enable unconjugated (free) bilirubin to become conjugated (bound) and safely excreted from the neonate via the urine and faeces. However, the neonatal liver is still maturing and the mechanism of bilirubin metabolism depends on a healthy infant who is feeding adequately. Factors that can adversely affect bilirubin metabolism are highlighted in Table 12.1.

Presentation and management

Physiological jaundice usually appears around day 3–4 and then fades over the next 10 days. Stools and urine should be of a normal colour and the baby feeds, demonstrates normal posture/movement and responsiveness. A healthy asymptomatic neonate does not usually require treatment. It is also important to consider parental skin colour and observe the baby in good natural light as yellow–green clothing, bedding and window coverings can make a baby appear jaundiced even when he/she is not.

Neonatal jaundice follows a cephalopedal colour progression (head, upper torso, lower torso, arms/legs, hands and feet). A transcutatneous bilirubinometer (TcB) can be used to measure the bilirubin level in babies whose gestational age is ≥35 weeks and who are over 24 hours of age. If a TcB is unavailable or the measurement indicates a bilirubin level >250 µmmol/L (lower limits may apply locally), a total serum bilirubin (TSB) test should be carried out to check the result. The neonate must be referred to the neonatologist for decisions regarding treatment and further investigation as to cause. The TSB result must be recorded on a TSB chart that is appropriate for the gestational age of the neonate.

The older method of detecting jaundice – Kramer's Rule (Kramer, 1969), whereby the skin of the infant is depressed with the examiner's finger at five bodily sites and the resulting blanched area assessed for colour – can prove to be an ineffectual visual method of assessing jaundice on non-white neonates.

Parents need to be aware of the positive actions that they can take to assist the physiological process of bilirubin metabolism and the possible negative changes to observe in their baby's general health that may indicate that the level of jaundice is increasing as a result of pathological causes (Table 12.2). They should always be told how to contact their healthcare professional in the event of any concern or negative changes in their baby's behaviour or colour so that urgent referral for assessment and/or treatment can be expedited.

Urgent referral to the paediatric team for assessment and TSB must always occur in the event of jaundice developing within 24 hours of birth and also if at any time a neonate appears to be significantly jaundiced and lethargic or dehydrated. The same action applies in the case of jaundice developing after 7 days or remaining after 14 days when causation has not been identified in an otherwise well (asymptomatic) baby.

Breastfeeding jaundice

Jaundice can present at 3–4 days or later, usually up to day 10 but can, in 15% of cases, continue beyond 2 weeks of age. The action of gluconeryl transferase is inhibited by hormones in breastmilk and further breastmilk hormones can cause conjugated bilirubin to revert to an unconjugated state. Slow bacterial colonisation of the gut because of the relatively low volume of milk that the baby imbibes during the first 3 days also exacerbates this process. Breastfeeding support may be necessary. If earlier initiation of breastfeeding has been problematic, continued support would prove beneficial and confidence building.

However, if the baby appears well and is feeding, even if having to be woken to do so, parents should be reassured and encouraged to feed their baby frequently. They should be encouraged not to stop breastfeeding or offer supplementary feeds (Clarke, 2013).

13 Pathological jaundice

Table 13.1 Factors that adversely affect bilirubin metabolism.

Factor	Effect
Increased haemolysis	Can lead to excessive bilirubin levels – possible causes include haemolytic disease of the newborn and maternal drug therapy (e.g. sulphonamides)
Shortage of albumin	Albumin is needed to bind with unconjugated fat-soluble bilirubin; may be caused by low serum albumin levels, asphyxia, acidosis, infection, hypoglycaemia and prematurity Particular drugs (e.g. sulphonamides and sodium benzoate) can also bind with albumin and compete with bilirubin
Hypoxia and hypoglycaemia	Both reduce the level of metabolism as both O_2 and glucose are necessary for the process to work. Glucose is the raw material used for the production of glucuronic acid
Low levels of gut bacteria and reduced peristalsis	Low levels of gut bacteria are normal at birth. Feeding encourages the population of normal fauna and flora in the neonatal gut and stimulates peristalsis. Slow of delayed initiation of feeding provides the circumstances that allow conjugated bilirubin to deconjugate (via action of β-glucuronidase) and re-enter the hepatic circulation

Table 13.2 Possible causes of unconjugated and conjugated jaundice.

Possible causes of unconjugated jaundice	
Day 1	Haemolytic disease of the newborn
Days 2–5	Haemolytic disease of the newborn; jaundice of prematurity; sepsis; extravascular blood; spherocytosis; polycythaemia and G6PD
Days 5–10	Sepsis; galactosaemia, hypothyroidism; drugs and breastmilk jaundice
Day 10+	Sepsis and urinary tract infection
Possible causes of conjugated jaundice	
Day 1–10	Neonatal hepatitis; rubella; CMV and syphilis
Day 10+	*Biliary obstruction* causes what is termed as obstructive jaundice, whereby the flow of bile is prevented from flowing into the intestine allowing a quantity of bilirubin to escape back into the bloodstream

CMV, cytomegalovius; G6PD, glucose-6-phosphate dehydrogenase deficiency.

Table 13.3 Urgent referral or admission for neonatal assessment.

Time period	Criteria for referral/admission
Within 2 hours	Jaundice in the first 24 hours of life
Within 6 hours	Jaundice first appears at more than 7 days of age
	Neonate is unwell (e.g. lethargy, fever, vomiting, irritability)
	Gestational age <35 weeks
	Prolonged jaundice: • Gestational age <37 weeks + jaundice for >21 days • Gestational age of ≥37 weeks + jaundice for >14 days
	Poor feeding and/or concerns re weight, particularly if breastfed
	Pale stools and dark urine

Table 13.4 Further investigations.

Investigation	Finding	Possible cause
Full blood count and blood film	↑ or ↓ white blood cell count or thrombocytopenia	Sepsis
	Haematocrit <45%	Haemolytic anaemia
	↑ Reticulocyte count	Haemolysis
Blood group and rhesus factor (mother and baby)	Maternal blood group O/baby blood group A or B	ABO incompatability
	Mother rhesus negative/baby rhesus positive	Rhesus isoimmunisation
Liver function tests	Increased liver enzymes	Congenital infection
Blood G6PD levels	Presence of G6PD – usually only taken in relation to ethnicity and gender	

Physical Examination of the Newborn at a Glance, First Edition. Denise (Dee) Campbell and Lyn Dolby.
© 2018 John Wiley & Sons, Ltd. Published 2018 by John Wiley & Sons, Ltd.

Necessity for bilirubin metabolism

As can be seen in Chapter 12, the process of bilirubin metabolism is complicated and dependent on a number of factors to enable unconjugated bilirubin to become conjugated and safely excreted from the neonate via the urine and faeces. Factors that can adversely affect bilirubin metabolism are highlighted in Table 13.1. Professional vigilance in observing for risk factors within the maternal and neonatal documentation and continual assessment of the baby's colour and well-being are vitally important for best practice. This is particularly important in the event that physiological and pathological jaundice occur together, for example prolonged jaundice may include breastfeeding jaundice, a normally occurring physiological condition that could mask something more serious such as biliary atresia.

Usually, physiological jaundice is harmless and is not an indication of an underlying disease or *pathology*. In 'physiological' jaundice, the aim is to prevent the level of jaundice from becoming more severe. The aim in 'pathological' jaundice is not only to prevent the level of bilirubin from rising further, but also to diagnose and treat the underlying cause(s) in order to prevent ongoing hyperbilirubinaemia (NICE, 2016).

The concern with hyperbilirubinaemia is that if it has a high affinity to fatty tissue and brain. Elevated levels of unconjugated bilirubin deposited in the neurons of the brain are neurotoxic and can cause acute or chronic encephalopathy. Kernicterus, or bilirubin encephalopathy, is a condition caused by bilirubin toxicity to the basal ganglia and various brainstem nuclei. Therefore, healthcare professionals need to be aware of the risk factors that are associated with pathological jaundice.

Pathological risk factors

The causes of unconjugated and conjugated jaundice can be seen in Tables 13.2 and 13.3, respectively, indicating the usual neonatal age that a specific factor may appear or be detected. The factors that can cause pathological jaundice include those that directly cause haemolysis of the red blood cells (e.g. rhesus or ABO incompatibility); excessive bruising and extravascular blood leakage; sepsis; metabolic disorders (e.g. galactosaemia, hereditary fructose intolerance, hypothyroidism, alpha-1 antitrypsin deficiency); Gilbert's syndrome and Crigler–Najjar syndrome (which although rare are caused by liver enzyme anomalies); glucose-6-phosphate dehydrogenase (G6PD) deficiency (a familial enzyme deficiency most common in Mediterranean, Middle Eastern, South-East Asian and African populations) and malformation or congenital obstruction of the biliary system such as biliary atresia (conjugated hyperbilirubinaemia arising from obstructive jaundice).

Assessment

Assessment during the first 48 hours is paramount if there is a history of possible risk factors. The parents should be asked if the baby's siblings or close family relatives experienced neonatal jaundice that required hospital treatment such as phototherapy or exchange blood transfusion. Investigate the ability of the baby to feed or if he/she is hard to wake and the daily number of wet and dirty nappies and colour of urine and stools. Check for signs of illness or fever, evidence of new or increased bleeding or bruising.

Always assess the baby's colour in bright (preferably natural) light at every contact opportunity within the first 72 hours of birth. Evaluate the colour of the whole body, noting any colour change in the sclerae, gums or palate or when pressing lightly on the nose (Queensland Maternity and Neonatal Clinical Guidelines Programme, 2012). A visual assessment of jaundice such as cephalocaudal progression or Kramer's zones is only a preliminary guide, and should not be used to estimate the level of bilirubin (NICE, 2016). Any adverse findings should instigate direct referral to a neonatologist, particularly if assessment of colour is difficult as in babies with darker skin coloration (NICE, 2016).

Serum bilirubin estimation and neonatal assessment

Any baby that is suspected or demonstrates obvious jaundice requires urgent assessment of their serum bilirubin (SBR). During the first 24 hours of life this assessment should occur within 2 hours, or in the case of a baby identified in Table 13.4, within 6 hours. SBR assessment enables confirmation of diagnosis and guides treatment according to national and local treatment thresholds.

The SBR should be plotted on a postnatal age-appropriate SBR chart according to the local threshold tables and treatment threshold graphs. The SBR level will need to be re-assessed every 6 hours until the level is below the treatment threshold, stable or falling.

Use of a transcutaneous bilirubinometer

In the past, an icterometer was used to measure bilirubin levels but it is now considered too inaccurate for such assessment and should not be used (NICE, 2016).

If a baby is over 24 hours of age and is ≥35 weeks gestational age, a transcutaneous bilirubinometer (TcB) can be used to measure the bilirubin level. However, if a TcB is not available, the SBR must be measured instead. For a TcB measurement indicating a bilirubin level >250 µmol/L, the SBR must be measured in order to check the result. The SBR should then be used if the bilirubin level is at or above the relevant treatment thresholds for the baby's gestational age and for all subsequent measurements (NICE, 2016).

Further investigations

In order to detect underlying causes, further investigations such as those in Table 13.4 should be conducted. However, investigations also include umbilical cord blood direct antiglobulin test (DAT; Coombs' test), although this should only be used to diagnose ABO or rhesus isoimmunisation and not to predict significant hyperbilirubinaemia (NICE, 2016). Microbiological cultures in relation to blood, urine and cerebrospinal fluid may also be investigated if infection is suspected but the source of the infection is unclear.

Treatment of choice

Treatment depends on the SBR level and/or cause of the jaundice. Therefore, appropriate treatment will be given to a baby with an underlying illness such as an infection. Phototherapy will be used if the SBR is at or above the treatment threshold in order to assist the conversion of unconjugated bilirubin into products that can be more easily excreted from the body via the stools and urine. An exchange transfusion is required in a baby with signs of bilirubin encephalopathy and who may be at risk of kernicterus or if the baby is not responding to phototherapy. If the underlying cause for jaundice is a condition such as biliary atresia then early admission for surgery will be the appropriate treatment of choice.

Parental support

Parents require a great deal of support from the moment the baby becomes visibly jaundiced or sleepy and reluctant to feed until the jaundice is resolved and any underlying cause treated. For some parents, this latter point may not be resolved easily or without further anxiety (e.g. G6PD). Discussion with parents needs to be clear, concise and in a language and terminology that they can understand. In some case, directing them to groups or associations will assist in the ongoing support that they may need.

Jaundice in the newborn should never be underestimated.

14 Metabolic disorders

Figure 14.1 Early signs and symptoms of metabolic disorder, showing deterioration pattern if untreated (some or all of the features may present).

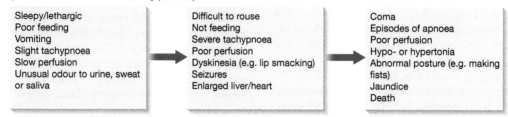

Sleepy/lethargic Poor feeding Vomiting Slight tachypnoea Slow perfusion Unusual odour to urine, sweat or saliva	Difficult to rouse Not feeding Severe tachypnoea Poor perfusion Dyskinesia (e.g. lip smacking) Seizures Enlarged liver/heart	Coma Episodes of apnoea Poor perfusion Hypo- or hypertonia Abnormal posture (e.g. making fists) Jaundice Death

Figure 14.2 Recessive inheritance (e.g. cystic fibrosis, Tay–Sachs disease).

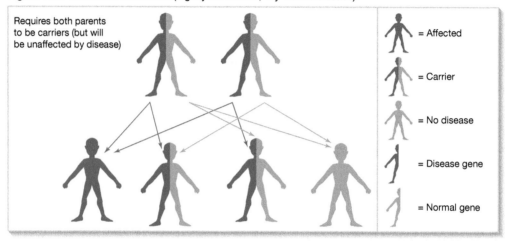

Requires both parents to be carriers (but will be unaffected by disease)

= Affected
= Carrier
= No disease
= Disease gene
= Normal gene

Figure 14.3 Dominant inheritance (e.g. diabetes mellitus type 1).

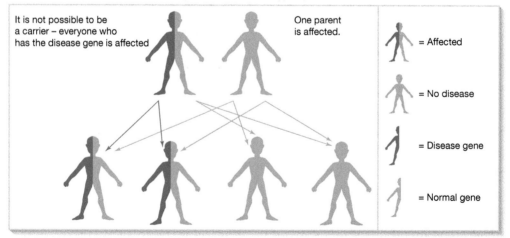

It is not possible to be a carrier – everyone who has the disease gene is affected

One parent is affected.

= Affected
= No disease
= Disease gene
= Normal gene

Physical Examination of the Newborn at a Glance, First Edition. Denise (Dee) Campbell and Lyn Dolby.
© 2018 John Wiley & Sons, Ltd. Published 2018 by John Wiley & Sons, Ltd.

This chapter aims to increase understanding of metabolic disorders in the newborn. There are known to be hundreds of genetic metabolic disorders, as they can result from even the most basic mutation of a gene. It will not be possible to cover them all so the aim here is to raise awareness generally and to mention some of the most common disorders. This chapter should be read in conjunction with Chapter 11 and having considered the associated risk factors.

What are metabolic disorders?

Metabolic disorders are a failure in the normal enzyme process of breaking down and converting ingested food into the many essential proteins and amino acids needed for normal body function. This may result in either too much or too little of these end products of metabolism. Too much, and the body has to store them in the liver, body fat or muscle, where excess levels can become toxic and damage cells. Too little, and the cells requiring these essential substances cannot work normally, leading to failures in whole body systems.

Causes of metabolic disorders

In the majority of metabolic disorders in the newborn, a mutated gene is responsible and will have caused the following:

• A deficiency in an enzyme or compound required for metabolism to take place – the most common cause of a metabolic disorder.
• A genetic disorder of (or damage to) any of the organs involved in metabolism (e.g. liver or pancreas).
• An abnormal chemical reaction that occurs during metabolism.

It is also possible for a vitamin or mineral deficiency, or excess, in the diet to cause a metabolic disorder. A problem of diet is rare in the newborn because of breastfeeding and, when bottle feeding, the use of specially formulated artificial feeds. However, it could occur in situations where inappropriate or incorrect artificial feeds are being given or if a breastfeeding mother has a severely deficient diet.

Types of congenital metabolic disorders

There are believed to be 800–1000 types of congenital metabolic disorders. The numbers and varieties make classification a challenge. Very simply, they can be seen to fall within four main categories.

1 **Disorders of metabolism** – deficiency of the enzymes required for synthesis of:
  • Carbohydrates (diabetes, galactosaemia);
  • Amino acids (phenylketonuria, maple syrup disease, isovaleric acidaemia, glutaric aciduria type 1, homocysteinuria);
  • Metal (Wilson's disease);
  • Steroids (congenital adrenal hyperplasia);
  • Fatty acids (medium chain acyl-coenzyme A dehydrogenase deficiency, MCADD).
2 **Disorders of the urea cycle** – deficiency of one of six enzymes required for removal of waste products (carbamoyl phosphate synthetase 1).
3 **Disorders of mitochondrial function** – dysfunction of cells to convert foods into the energy they need (Kearns–Sayre syndrome).
4 **Disorders specific to lysosomal or peroxisomal storage** – deficiency or absence of the enzymes that break down toxins within cell spaces (Zellweger's syndrome, Gaucher's disease, Tay–Sachs disease, cystic fibrosis).

Signs and symptoms

These are dependent on the exact type of disorder, disease or syndrome. Presentation at birth can be as extreme as hydrops fetalis (Gaucher's disease) or dysmorphic features (Zellweger's syndrome). In most cases there will be no signs at birth; then, a gradual onset of neurological symptoms, metabolic acidosis and/or hypoglycaemia. Progression leads to possible cardiac disease; liver dysfunction; bone damage; central nervous system (CNS) damage; and death.

Routine screening in the early newborn period can detect a number of disorders before significant symptoms or harm occur. Detection otherwise may be signs of the earliest onset and deterioration pattern which begins with the sleepy baby, feeding problems and failure to thrive (Figure 14.1).

Principles of treatment

These conditions cannot be cured but instead must be managed to limit damaging side effects. The three main principles engaged are as follow:

1 Alteration of the diet to remove, or prevent the introduction of, any foods that cannot be digested.
2 The introduction of enzymes or supplements to correct any imbalance.
3 Treatment to remove or reduce any toxic substances.

Most common congenital metabolic disorders

All of the individual conditions are relatively rare but, as so many exist, the chance of a newborn baby having one of the disorders increases. It is likely that all maternity unit based practitioners will come across a metabolic disorder at least once in their careers. Those based in the community or involved in longer term care will meet them more frequently. The more common disorders are as follow:

• **Congenital adrenal hyperplasia** – typically, the adrenal glands produce insufficient cortisol and too much androgen; may result in ambiguous genitalia.
• **Cystic fibrosis** – recessive inherited disorder (Figure 14.2) affecting exocrine glands; sodium and chlorine excess in cells cause dehydrated, thickened mucus secretions in lung cells.
• **Diabetes mellitus** – may be type 1 (insulin dependent) or type 2 resulting from genetic factors (Figure 14.3) or uncontrolled maternal diabetes including gestational forms.
• **Galactosaemia** – inability to break down galactose to glucose.
• **Gaucher's disease** – an excess of glucosylceramide; more severe forms affect the nervous system. Most common inherited genetic condition for Ashkenazi Jews.
• **Maple syrup disease** – inability to break down certain amino acids; severity ranges from mild to severe (when brain damage can occur). So named because of the sweet maple smell of the urine.
• **MCADD** – inability to break down medium-chain fatty acids into acetyl-CoA; symptoms include hypoglycaemia and sudden death.
• **Phenylketonuria (PKU)** – inability to break down phenylalanine; build up in the blood and brain.
• **Tay–Sachs disease** – gangliosides accumulate in the brain causing progressive damage from 7 months; death by age 4 years.
• **Wilson's disease** – the body is unable to remove excess copper storage – mainly in the brain and liver.
• **Zellweger's syndrome** – life-threatening, multi-system failure to break down toxins. Facial and skeletal dysmorphia are often present.

15 Jitteriness, seizures and hypotonia

Box 15.1 Signs of subtle neonatal seizures.

- Staring, locked eye position
- Eyes contracted to one side
- Lip smacking movements
- Sucking lower lip
- Sucking tongue
- Pedalling legs
- Swimming movements of upper and/or lower limbs
- Apnoea

EEG required to confirm seizure

Box 15.2 Types of neonatal seizures.

- **Clonic** – rhythmic jerking of a small area (tongue, face, diaphragm) or large area (limb, head)
- **Tonic** – sustained muscle contraction; symmetrical or asymmetrical
- **Myoclonic** – arrhythmic jerking; single, rapid, repetitive; small area (finger) or whole body; may mimic Moro reflex

These can also be:

- Focal
- Multifocal
- Generalised

Table 15.1 Distinguishing jitteriness from seizures.
Source: Sinha *et al.* (2012). Reproduced with permission of John Wiley & Sons.

	Jitteriness	Convulsions
Stimulus provoked	Yes	No
Predominant movement	Rapid, oscillatory	Clonic, tonic
Movements cease when limb is held	Yes	No
Conscious state	Awake or asleep	Altered
Eye deviation	No	Yes

Table 15.2 Causes of neonatal seizures, indicating time of onset and frequency (+).
Source: Sinha *et al.* (2012). Reproduced with permission of John Wiley & Sons.

	Time of onset and relative frequency	
	0–2 days	2–10 days
Asphyxia	+++	–
Neonatal/perinatal stroke	+++	+
Intracranial haemorrhage	++	+
Hypocalcaemia	++	+
Hypoglycaemia	++	+
Infection	+	++
Developmental abnormalities	+	+
Drug withdrawal	+	
Inborn errors of metabolism	+	+
Pyridoxine deficiency	++	

Table 15.3 Causes of newborn hypotonia.
Source: Sinha *et al.* (2012). Reproduced with permission of John Wiley & Sons.

Paralytic	Non-paralytic
Spinal muscular atrophy (Werdnig–Hoffmann)	Birth asphyxia
Congenital muscular dystrophy	Down's syndrome
Congenital myopathy	Prader–Willi syndrome
Congenital myotonic dystrophy	Skeletal and connective tissue disorders
Myasthenia gravis	Drugs
	Benign congenital hypotonia

Physical Examination of the Newborn at a Glance, First Edition. Denise (Dee) Campbell and Lyn Dolby.
© 2018 John Wiley & Sons, Ltd. Published 2018 by John Wiley & Sons, Ltd.

This chapter looks at a number of symptoms associated with newborn disorders that can complicate the physical examination. It should be read in conjunction with other relevant chapters such as those related to infection, neurological (head and spine), cardiovascular and metabolic disorders. The practitioner must be able to differentiate between physiological and pathological changes in body movements and tone. This will enable appropriate referral, without delay. Appreciation of the differing causes, management and prognoses will support effective communication both when referring and between parents and carers. The symptoms are all relatively common but are often missed, misinterpreted or misdiagnosed (Table 15.1).

Jitteriness

Jitteriness is a fast intermittent tremor that mostly affects the limbs but less noticeably can affect the face and body. It results from excessive neuromuscular activity and the immaturity of the nervous system and can be deliberately stimulated. In the majority of cases it is not associated with abnormality but is an over-active response to stimuli. Although more common with premature babies, it still occurs in around half of term newborns. Most often stopping within days, it can continue for months even when there is no pathological cause.

The Moro reflex may be mistaken for jitteriness. Twitching during sleep can also sometimes be described as jitteriness by parents but these asymmetrical movements are normal during sleep and are only a concern if prolonged or cyanosis is observed.

To confirm that an episode is jitteriness (and not any other pathological body movement), the examiner should try holding a limb (gently but firmly) and flexing the joint. If the tremor stops it is not any other form of seizure. It may also stop during sucking so the sucking reflex can be stimulated and the tremor observed. The jitteriness should appear:

- Symmetrically across the two sides of the body, never one-sided;
- Rhythmical and gentle, with no major jumping movement of the limbs;
- Without unusual eye, mouth or limb movements (Box 15.1);
- Without breathing pattern or heart rate changes.

Confirmation that this is jitteriness (and not a seizure) does not automatically rule out complications. If this is an otherwise healthy newborn who is feeding well, and it was a brief episode and not re-occurring, then no further investigations are required. However, if there are risk factors or the jitteriness is frequent and persistent, referral and further investigations are needed. There are a number of conditions that are associated with pathological jitteriness:

- Asphyxia;
- Hypernatraemia;
- Hypocalcaemia;
- Hypoglycaemia (this is the most common cause);
- Hypomagnesaemia;
- Intracranial haemorrhage;
- Sepsis;
- Withdrawal from maternal drugs (fetal abstinence syndrome).

Seizures (convulsions or fits)

Electrical impulses within the brain can become over- or under-active when a chemical imbalance occurs. A clinically apparent change in movement or tone occurs as a result and this is known as a seizure. The most common causes of early onset seizures are associated with episodes of asphyxia or stroke; later onset seizures are more commonly associated with severe sepsis (e.g. meningitis, encephalitis; Sinha *et al.*, 2012; Table 15.2). Seizures remain the most common symptom of neurological damage in infancy and are associated with disability and mortality (Vasudevan and Levene, 2013). It is important to appreciate that not all seizures are epilepsy. In epilepsy, seizures are not provoked by an acute cause (Hart *et al.*, 2015).

The most common seizures during the first 6 weeks of life are subtle seizures, where the clinical signs are often minor and frequently missed or confused for signs of hunger (Box 15.1). Equally, it should be remembered that these signs can be seen even alongside generalised tonic movements, without EEG changes and therefore not confirmed as seizures. The other main seizures possible (Box 15.2) may be accompanied by heart rate, respiration rate or blood pressure changes, as well as salivation and pupil changes. They can last for as little as 10 s to a number of minutes and come in quick succession or be minutes apart. After the subtle seizure, clonic and myoclonic seizures are more likely. Tonic seizures are more rare but carry the poorest prognosis as they are associated with an increased likelihood of cerebral haemorrhage (Hart *et al.*, 2015).

Benign neonatal sleep myoclonus (Cross, 2013)

This is a benign myoclonus that only happens during sleep. Movements involve some or all limbs but not the face; are bilateral and repetitive; and resolve by 4 months without lasting side effects.

Hyperekplexia or startle disease (Cross, 2013)

This is a genetically inherited, autosomal condition, characterised by excessive startle, generalised muscle rigidity and possible tonic spasm. Intubation may be required to prevent hypoxia, and sudden infant death syndrome is high risk. Events can be triggered by unexpected sounds or sensations – even a tap on the nose.

Hypotonia (floppiness)

This occurs when the newborn demonstrates a lack of muscle tone. This can be to varying degrees: localised (facial or Erb's palsy) or generalised (frog position); with or without evidence of muscle weakness. Tone decreases with degrees of prematurity but hypotonia is always abnormal in a term infant. The damage may be to the central or peripheral nervous system (e.g. asphyxia, trauma); muscles (e.g. congenital dystrophy); or a neuromuscular junction (e.g. myasthenia gravis; Sinha *et al.*, 2012; Table 15.3). The condition may be temporary (e.g. metabolic or electrolyte disorder) or permanent (chromosomal condition or cerebral damage). Occasionally, a condition can be associated with both seizures and hypotonia (hypoxic–ischaemic encephalopathy).

16 Congenital infection and sepsis

Table 16.1 Infections and their side effects.

Infection risk	Most common possible side effects for the newborn
Candida albicans	Coated tongue and gums (white, creamy plaque), nappy rash
Cytomegalovirus	Microcephaly, hydrocephaly, cataract, chorioretinitis, hearing loss, organ disease, cerebral palsy, delayed development, brain calcification, rash (blueberry muffin spots)
Group B streptococcus	Septicaemia, pneumonia, meningitis, blindness, deafness, learning disability, lung weakness or even death
Herpes simplex	Petechiae, infectious pustules, blisters and scarring, chorioretinitis, liver defects, anaemia, thrombocytopenia
Human immunodeficiency virus	Intra-uterine growth retardation, microcephaly, facial defects (prominent forehead, triangular philtrum, enlarged lips)
Meconium aspiration	Respiratory distress, cerebral irritability, pneumonitis, pneumothorax, hypoxia, acidosis, vascular necrosis, asphyxia or even death
Parvovirus B19	Slapped cheek facial rash, anaemia, eye defects, heart failure, hydrops fetalis
Rubella	Intra-uterine growth retardation, microcephaly, hydrocephaly, cataract, retinitis, glaucoma, deafness, heart defects, liver defects, hearing loss, rash (blueberry muffin spots), anaemia, bone weakness
Gonorrhoea Chlamydia	Conjunctivitis, profusely discharging eyes (ophthalmia)
Staphylococcus aureus	Yellow spots on skin, omphalitis, paronychia
Syphilis	Intra-uterine growth retardation, excoriating rash on palms of hands and soles of feet, changes in bone growth or development
Toxoplasmosis	Intra-uterine growth retardation, microcephaly, hydrocephaly, cataract, retinitis, deafness, heart defects, liver defects, hearing loss, rash, anaemia, brain calcification
Treponema pallidum	Hydrocephalus, deafness, bone defects, developmental defects
Varicella zoster (chickenpox)	Eye damage, microcephaly, defects in the brain or spine (causing hypoplasia or partial paralysis), skin excoriation and scarring, urogenital defects

The newborn is at risk from various sources of infection. These may be transplacental, ascending uterine, intrapartum, breastfeeding or via direct contact after birth. Whilst many maternal infections do not affect the fetus, the ones that do increase both morbidity and mortality through miscarriage, premature labour, growth retardation or development abnormalities. Any infection should be treated as significant because of the potential side effects and the possibility of a rapid decline in the health of the newborn. Infections must be managed without delay, including early (and possibly urgent) referral for full investigation and septic screen.

Risk factors

There are a number of maternal risk factors that will increase the risk of congenitally acquired infections. Some of these are routinely screened for in pregnancy whilst others may be screened for after identification of increased risk. The maternal history should be reviewed for evidence of any of the following:

- Viral infection (e.g. human immunodeficiency virus, rubella, cytomegalovirus, parvovirus, herpes simplex virus, varicella zoster virus);
- Sexually transmitted disease (e.g. syphilis, chlamydia, gonorrhoea);
- Bacterial infection (e.g. group B streptococcus);
- Fungal infection (e.g. *Candida albicans*);
- Maternal rash, malaise or 'flu like' symptoms;
- Antibodies detected during serology screening;
- Maternal pyrexia;
- Preterm and/or prolonged rupture of membranes;
- Meconium liquor;
- Chorioamnionitis;
- Substance misuse;
- Previous infant with group B streptococcus;
- Toxoplasmosis (parasite) screening.

Following birth, the sepsis risk is increased in the presence of the following:

- Maternal infection (e.g. mastitis);
- Inappropriate hygiene standards;
- Maternal learning disability (affecting hygiene standards);
- Exposure to infection from sibling, partner or visitor;
- Prematurity;
- Hospital delivery – environment, staff and equipment;
- Invasive procedures (and prolonged labour).

Signs and symptoms

Information should be gleaned from the patterns of sleeping, feeding and if there has been any vomiting. This should reveal the following:

- Any unusual drowsiness or an unresponsive baby;
- Infrequent or poor feeding;
- Poor weight gain (at the 6 week examination);
- Vomiting.

In addition, the practitioner should look for signs of the following:

- Tachypnoea, bradypnoea, chest recession, grunting or apnoea (often a first or early sign of sepsis);
- Abnormalities linked to congenital infections (Table 16.1);
- Haematuria (ensure this is not pseudo-menstruation or urates);
- Inflammation, redness or an area of localised heat;

- Pallor or a mottled appearance;
- Delayed perfusion (poor capillary refill time);
- Localised serous fluid leak, septic spots or any purulent exudate;
- Diarrhoea or dehydration;
- Systemic temperature that is low, raised (above 38°C) or unstable;
- High-pitched cry;
- Hypotonia or hypertonia, jitteriness or seizures;
- Hypo- or hyperglycaemia;
- An area of swelling and/or tenderness;
- Bradycardia or tachycardia;
- Jaundice or enlarged liver;
- Acidosis or shock.

Management

Any high risk or symptomatic newborn should be managed accordingly. The practitioner must review the results of any of the following:

- Regular observations of respiration efforts, temperature, heart rate, colour, behaviour, responsiveness and oxygen saturation. The Newborn Early Warning Trigger and Track (NEWTT) risk identification and observational chart (British Association of Perinatal Medicine, 2015) complements clinical skills.
- Septic screen (swabs; urine, blood or stool samples; or, cerebrospinal fluid from lumbar puncture).
- Monitoring of fluid balance including feeding and excretion.

Where significant sepsis has been confirmed, antibiotic treatment and admission to a neonatal intensive care unit (NICU) will have been likely for respiratory and cardiovascular support; thermoregulation; fluid/feed supplementation; medications; and 24 hour monitoring.

Group B streptococcus

This is the most common cause of newborn sepsis and has the potential to be fatal. This bacteria can colonise the maternal vaginal tract and introduce the risk of both ascending infection (during prolonged rupture of the membranes) and contact during delivery. It can also be passed in breastmilk or by a carer. Preventative management includes intrapartum antibiotics (at least 2 hours before delivery), followed by regular observation of the newborn to include respiration and temperature monitoring. Unmanaged, the risks to the newborn are as follow:

- Respiratory distress and/or pneumonia;
- Septicaemia;
- Meningitis.

These can progress to a longer term blindness, deafness, learning disability, lung weakness or even death.

Conjunctivitis

Redness of the conjunctiva, purulent discharge and oedema are strong indicators of infection. The most common causes relate to a blocked lacrimal duct, *Staphylococcus aureus* or contact with a sexually transmitted infection during delivery. Of greatest concern is the ophthalmia identified at the first examination caused by *Neisseria gonorrhoeae* (occurring within 24 hours of birth) which can cause permanent scarring if management is delayed. Chlamydial and syphilitic infections typically present later than the first examination.

17 Anaemia and polycythaemia

Figure 17.1 Fetal cells – anaemia.
Source: Lissauer and Fanaroff (2011). Reproduced with permission of John Wiley & Sons.

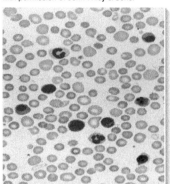

Figure 17.2 Maternal cells mixed with fetal haemaglobin.
Source: Lissauer and Fanaroff (2011). Reproduced with permission of John Wiley & Sons.

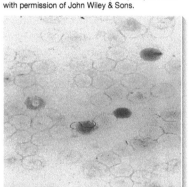

Fetomaternal hemorrhage. (Fig. 17.1) Anaemia (number of red cells are reduced), nucleated red cells (erythroblasts) and reticulocytes on a blood smear (film) from a term neonate with severe anaemia at birth (4.5 g/dL) caused by fetomaternal haemorrhage.

(Fig. 17.2) Kleihauer test on maternal blood from the same baby showing several intensely pink-stained cells containing HbF, which is resistant to acid lysis

Figure 17.3 Causes and investigations of anaemia – with and without jaundice complication.
Source: Lissauer and Fanaroff (2011). Reproduced with permission of John Wiley & Sons.

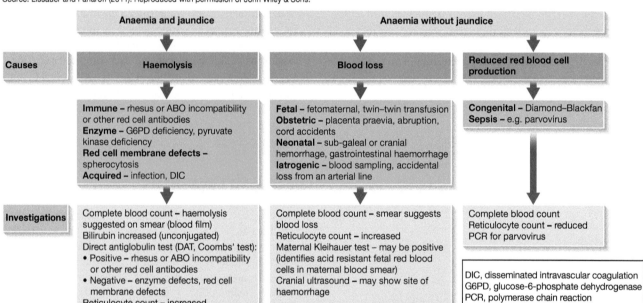

	Anaemia and jaundice	Anaemia without jaundice	
Causes	**Haemolysis**	**Blood loss**	**Reduced red blood cell production**
	Immune – rhesus or ABO incompatibility or other red cell antibodies **Enzyme** – G6PD deficiency, pyruvate kinase deficiency **Red cell membrane defects** – spherocytosis **Acquired** – infection, DIC	**Fetal** – fetomaternal, twin–twin transfusion **Obstetric** – placenta praevia, abruption, cord accidents **Neonatal** – sub-galeal or cranial hemorrhage, gastrointestinal haemorrhage **Iatrogenic** – blood sampling, accidental loss from an arterial line	**Congenital** – Diamond–Blackfan **Sepsis** – e.g. parvovirus
Investigations	Complete blood count – haemolysis suggested on smear (blood film) Bilirubin increased (unconjugated) Direct antiglobulin test (DAT, Coombs' test): • Positive – rhesus or ABO incompatibility or other red cell antibodies • Negative – enzyme defects, red cell membrane defects Reticulocyte count – increased	Complete blood count – smear suggests blood loss Reticulocyte count – increased Maternal Kleihauer test – may be positive (identifies acid resistant fetal red blood cells in maternal blood smear) Cranial ultrasound – may show site of haemorrhage	Complete blood count Reticulocyte count – reduced PCR for parvovirus

DIC, disseminated intravascular coagulation
G6PD, glucose-6-phosphate dehydrogenase
PCR, polymerase chain reaction

Figure 17.4 Oxygen affinity of neonatal haemoglobin versus adult haemoglobin.
Source: Lissauer and Fanaroff (2011). Reproduced with permission of John Wiley & Sons.

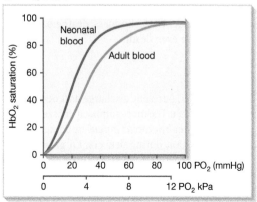

Figure 17.5 Plethoric newborn (nasogastric tube associated with poor feeding).
Source: Lissauer and Fanaroff (2011). Reproduced with permission of John Wiley & Sons.

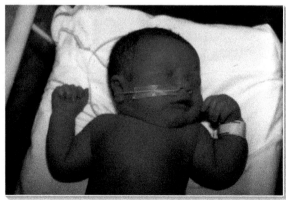

This chapter aims to help the examiner understand anaemia and polycythaemia: to enable recognition of risk factors, signs and symptoms. The most debated contributing factor for both conditions is delayed cord clamping.

Cord clamping

The blood volume of a newborn is in the range 75–100 mL/kg. Delayed cord clamping can increase this by as much as 25–30% with the benefit of reducing the likelihood of both physiological and iron deficiency anaemia. However, the increased circulating blood volume and potential concentration of red blood cells can also increase the risk of polycythaemia and jaundice. The Resuscitation Council (UK) (2015) guidelines recommend delaying cord clamping for at least 1 minute for all healthy newborn infants and for up to 3 minutes for premature births. This assumes resuscitation is not required and maternal consent has been given.

Anaemia

Neonatal anaemia is defined by the reduced level of circulating haemoglobin (Figure 17.1). Haemoglobin consists of red pigmented haem (containing ferrous iron) and the protein globin. It performs the essential role of transporting oxygen around the various cells of the body. Lower levels of circulating oxygen in utero necessitate a high fetal haemoglobin level and higher oxygen affinity (Figure 17.4). This remains high for the neonate, with a normal range of 150–230 g/L. Below 100 g/L is considered to be anaemia and below 80 g/L is considered severe. Anaemia can occur in either of the following situations:

- **Haemorrhage** –in utero, at or after birth;
- **Reduction in red cells** – under-production or excessive destruction (Figure 17.3).

Predisposing factors

Ironically, the most common anaemia is induced through repeated blood sampling from premature infants. Other factors associated with haemorrhage include the following:

- **Placental trauma** – abruption, praevia, chorionic villi sampling, trauma during surgery, vasa praevia, snapped cord;
- **Fetomaternal transfusion** – evidence of raised Kleihauer test (Figure 17.2);
- **Twin–twin transfusion** – one twin anaemic, the other polycythaemic;
- **Birth trauma** – fracture, bruising, cephalhaematoma, subgaleal haematoma, abdominal or chest compression;
- **Abnormality** – gastrointestinal bleeding.

Physiological reduction of the haemoglobin occurs naturally after birth to reduce the high level inherited from fetal life. Pathological destruction, under-production and abnormalities in formation are also possible associated with the following risk factors:

- **Uterine hypoxia** – meconium in utero, sinusoidal fetal heart, fetal blood gases, fetal compromise;
- **Placental insufficiency** – growth-deficient fetus or newborn;
- **Maternal disease** – diabetes, disseminated intravascular coagulation, autoimmune disease;
- **Congenital infection;**
- **Haemolysis** – rhesus or ABO incompatibility (antibodies, positive Coombs' test), sibling anaemia;

- **Genetic disease** – Diamond–Blackfan, glucose-6-phosphate dehydrogenase (G6PD) deficiency, thalassaemia;
- **Blood cell disorders** – pyknocytosis, spherocytosis;
- **Dietary deficiency** – vitamin E or iron;
- **Hormone imbalance** – reduction in, or lack of erythropoietin.

Most common early signs and symptoms

- Pale;
- Lethargic;
- Poor feeding or failure to thrive;
- Tachycardia;
- Tachypnoea (deteriorating to intermittent apnoea);
- Enlarged liver;
- Jaundice.

Polycythaemia

This is a condition of excessive red blood cells or high packed cell volume (haematocrit). The percentage of packed cells to whole blood at birth is in the range 55–68%, peaking at 6–12 hours because of haemoconcentration. Polycythaemia is relatively common at levels above 65%. The normal range by the 6 week examination has dropped to 32–45%. Polycythaemia does not automatically mean that blood becomes viscous but this will complicate almost half of cases and associated microthrombi may develop and block smaller blood vessels. Polycythaemia is associated with the following conditions:

- Increased red cell production (erythropoietin);
- Increased blood volume.

Predisposing factors

- **Hypoxic episodes stimulate compensatory red cell increase for oxygen-carrying capacity** – placental abruption, maternal smoker, placental insufficiency, poor fetal growth, post date pregnancy.
- **Excessive placental transfusion** – delayed cord clamping, twin–twin transfusion, gravity (infant below placental height).
- **Maternal disease** – diabetic mother, gestational diabetes, pre-eclampsia, heart disease, renal disease.
- **Newborn disease** – endocrine abnormalities linked to fetal hypoxia (thyrotoxicosis, Beckwith–Wiedemann syndrome, hyperglycaemia).
- **Newborn genetic disorders** – trisomies 13, 18 or 21, diabetes.

Most common early signs and symptoms

Many polycythaemic newborns are asymptomatic but signs will increase according to the degree of problem:

- Normal colour at rest, deep red–purple when distressed (plethoric; Figure 17.5);
- Sleepiness and poor feeding;
- Irritability on handling;
- Oliguria and/or haematuria;
- Jitteriness and tremors, progressing to seizures;
- Thrombosis and cerebrovascular accidents;
- Tachypnoea (respiratory disease and intermittent apnoea);
- Cyanosis (rare as a neonate) – progressing to heart failure;
- Priapism (male infants);
- Hypo- or hyperglycaemia;
- Jaundice and hyperbilirubinaemia;
- Necrotising enterocolitis;
- Thrombocytopenia.

18 Intrapartum injury/trauma

Figure 18.1 Incidence of common types of birth injury.

Arrow denotes order of increasing incidence	
Cephalhaematoma	1 : 100
Facial nerve palsy	1 : 500
Brachial plexus injury	0.5–1 : 1000
Subaponeurotic haemorrhage (subgaleal)	1 : 1250
Major subdural haemorrhage	1 : 50 000
Skull fractures	Rare
Spinal cord injuries	Very rare

Figure 18.2 Areas of extracranial and intercranial haemorrhage.
Source: Adapted from Brozansky *et al*., (2012). Reproduced with permission of Elsevier.

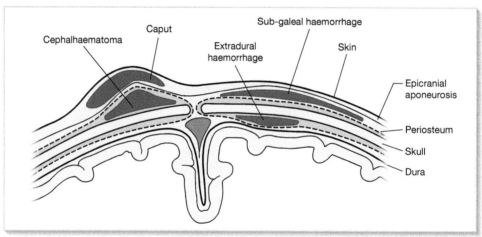

Table 18.1 Brachial plexus injury.

Cause	Excessive lateral flexion, rotation or traction of the neonatal neck at delivery Unexplained – possible prenatal cause
Erb's palsy	Where the arm lies adducted in the classic waiter's tip position but movement of the fingers is retained
Klumpke's palsy	More likely to occur in preterm infants during a difficult delivery of the head during a breech delivery It involves the small muscles of the hand with accompanying wrist drop and flaccid paralysis of the hand resulting in an absent grasp reflex
Total paralysis of the arm	Trauma has occurred to all trunks of the brachial plexus, resulting in flaccidity of the arm The cutis marmorata may be visible as a result of vasomotor disturbance In the event of bilateral impact, spinal injury should be suspected

At or soon after birth, particular minor abnormalities or birth injuries may be observed. Some may have occurred during the passage of the fetus through the bony pelvis, others may be the result of the instruments used during labour (e.g. amnihook, fetal scalp electrode, ventouse/forceps). On occasion, injury may have been sustained from excessive force or as the consequence of urgent actions performed during delivery (e.g. shoulder dystocia).

The incidence for the common birth injuries is given in Figure 18.1.

Soft tissue injury

Traumatic petechiae

Traumatic petechiae can be visualised from head to upper chest, usually as the result of a difficult delivery. Petechiae can be mistaken for cyanosis but O_2 saturation will be normal. They commonly occur with breech delivery or when the umbilical cord is wound tightly round the neonatal neck, resulting in a sudden increase in intrathoracic pressure as the chest compresses at

Physical Examination of the Newborn at a Glance, First Edition. Denise (Dee) Campbell and Lyn Dolby.
© 2018 John Wiley & Sons, Ltd. Published 2018 by John Wiley & Sons, Ltd.

delivery. Petechiae in this instance are transitory, usually fading within 2–3 days but should not be confused with generalised petechiae across the body which are associated with low platelets or coagulopathy.

Bruising
Bruising may result from precipitate or traumatic birth as the result of abnormal presentation (e.g. face, brow or breech) or in the presence of thrombocytopenia. Parents should be made aware that depending on the degree of bruising, jaundice may be more likely because of the increased bilirubin breakdown.

Subcutaneous fat necrosis
This is an obvious induration of the skin caused by pressure being applied to the skin (e.g. forceps blades to the face).

Extracranial trauma
Cephalhaematoma
Cephalhaematoma is the result of repeated contact between the fetal skull and the maternal pelvis, although pressure caused during vacuum delivery can also be a factor (Figure 18.2). Shearing of the veins between the periosteum and cranial bones (usually the parietal region but occasionally occipital) causes bleeding, the extent of which is limited by the suture lines. Gentle palpation of the area will assist in detecting any underlying skull fracture. The subperiosteal bleeding is slow and may not be visible until some hours or days later when it eventually reaches its fullest extent. Swelling may persist for several weeks. Parents should be made aware of the increased risk of jaundice.

Subaponeurotic (or subgaleal) haemorrhage
This condition is most often but not exclusively seen in black infants. This rare type of haemorrhage is the result of bleeding occurring beneath the aponeurotic sheet that joins the parts of the occipitofrontalis muscle. Causative factors include trauma during delivery (e.g. vacuum extraction) or may be the result of a coagulation disorder. Rapid swelling produces the 'hot water bottle' sign, where the scalp becomes fluctuant on touch. Blood loss can be acute and underestimated, with haemoglobin levels falling significantly, resulting in neonatal shock. Rapid diagnosis and management with fluid replacement (blood or volume expanders) is paramount (Colditz *et al.,* 2014).

Intercranial trauma
Haemorrhage
This may occur as a direct consequence of trauma, but is more often the result of hypoxic–ischaemic injury. Encephalopathy or seizures may be present and neonatal consultant management is required on recognition.

Bone and joint injuries
Skull fracture
A skull fracture may be associated with forceps delivery or, more rarely, head compression with the maternal sacral promontory. Linear fractures usually require no treatment but depressed or large fractures may indicate underlying trauma and neurosurgical consultation should be sought. Depressed skull fractures can take some months to resolve post birth.

Fractured clavicle
The clavicle is the most frequent bone to be fractured and is usually associated with shoulder dystocia or a difficult breech delivery. As with adults, management is minimal with the offer of pain relief if the baby appears uncomfortable (Wall *et al.,* 2014).

Fractured humerus or femur
Both occur rarely, usually as a result of trauma during delivery. Immobilisation is the care management of choice. Radial nerve injury can sometimes occur with the former and integrity of the nerve supply should be assessed.

Multiple fractures
The incidence of multiple fractures is rare and therefore the possibility of osteogenesis imperfecta should be explored.

Unusual fractures
Fractures occurring after birth or after the baby has been discharged home should always be investigated. Parents need to be cared for sensitively as the inference is often of a non-accidental injury. Provision of an accurate account from both the parents and the healthcare professionals at the time is paramount. If no immediate cause is clearly apparent, social services and the police are often involved. Reviewing and gaining an understanding of the safeguarding policies within one's own NHS Trust is invaluable.

Peripheral nerve trauma
Generally, the most likely nerve trauma to be found is the result of a *brachial plexus injury* which has a strong association with shoulder dystocia. However, it can also occur during delivery of the after-coming head in a breech presentation. The three types of paralysis are seen in Table 18.1.

Facial nerve palsy
Oblique application of forceps blades or prolonged pressure within the bony pelvis may result in an inability to close the eye and a lack of expression on the affected side when the baby cries. In most cases recovery occurs by 6 weeks of age.

Radial nerve trauma
Rarely seen in practice, but radial nerve trauma may result from a fracture of the humerus if there is difficulty in delivery of the arm during a breech delivery. Previously, the giving of an intramuscular injection into the deltoid region was associated with radial nerve damage which is why this area is now avoided for injection.

Other rarer forms of nerve trauma include *sciatic and phrenic nerve injury, recurrent laryngeal nerve* and *spinal cord injury.*

Organ injuries
Liver, spleen, kidneys and testes
A traumatic breech delivery (or, rarely, an atraumatic vertex delivery) can cause subcapsular haematoma of the liver. In the event of hepatosplenomegaly (rhesus haemolytic disease, diabetic mother), rupture of the liver or spleen may have already occurred. Rupture of the kidneys can also occur in preterm infants who present breech at delivery.

Adrenal haemorrhage may occur with breech deliveries, but an overwhelming bacterial infection of disseminated intravascular coagulopathy is most likely to be the cause. Bruising of the testes and haemorrhage may be seen in breech deliveries and are usually treated with analgesia.

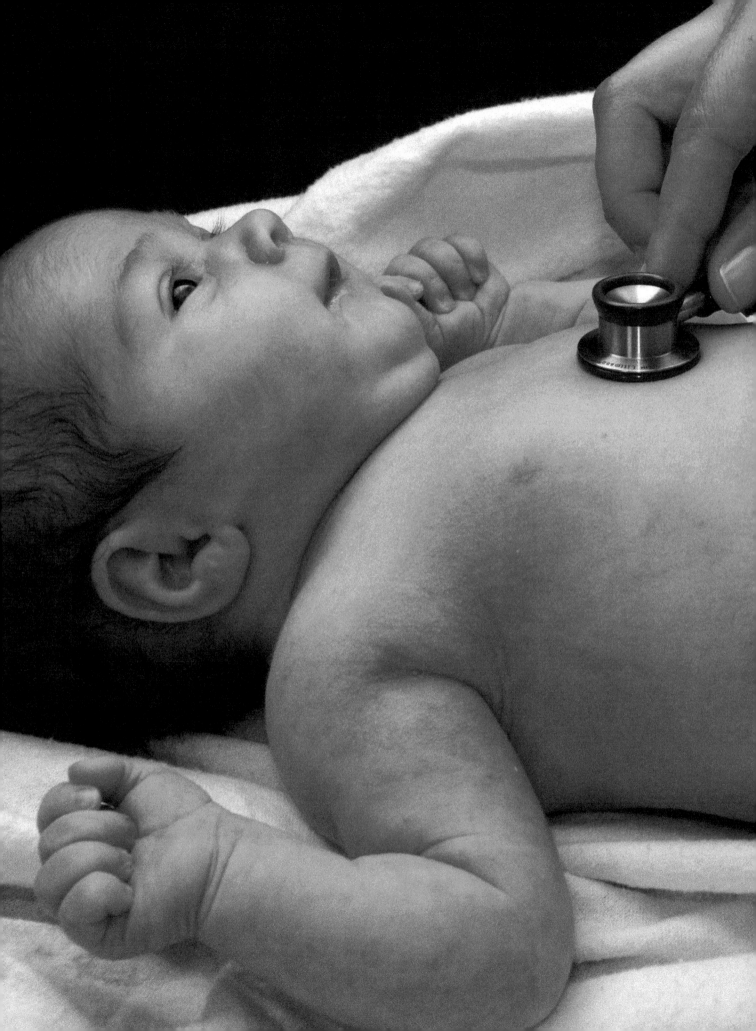

Allied assessments

Part 3

Chapters

19 Initial examination at birth – overview

Table 19.1 Key areas of assessment in the initial examination at birth.

Aspect	Observe and assess the following elements	
Colour	Pink/well perfused Jaundiced: predisposing factors, does the baby appear well?	
Head	Suture lines/integrity of skull bones Fontanelles: number, size, normal? Facial features: dysmorphia Ears: shape, size,	Head circumference: tape measure should be placed round widest part of the baby's head with the centimetre edge pointing towards the brow line
Neck/clavicles	Tumours, webbing, fractures	
Palate	Digital and visual inspection: teeth present? Evidence of tongue tie? Is the soft and hard palate complete?	
Posture/behaviour	Assess tone, good flexion, normal movements and responsiveness to speech, light and touch	
Heart rate	Normal apex beat = 100–160/min	
Respiratory	Normal respiratory rate = 30–60/min. Normal breathing movements with equal chest rise on both sides and no chest recession	
Chest	Normal shape, two nipples equally spaced. Presence of gynaecomastia?	
Abdomen	Normal 'pot-bellied' shape, smooth and no masses visible	
Umbilicus	Correct number of vessels in cord. Clamp on and secure. No visible sign of herniation	
Upper limbs	Count number of digits on left and right hands, by slightly separating each one as it is counted. Palm creases × 2 (if 1, is there any related familial history or any other dysmorphic features?) Check there is nothing hiding in the palms of the hands and for interdigital webbing. Check bone integrity, movement	
Lower limbs	Count number of digits on left and right foot, by slightly separating each one as it is counted, and check for interdigital webbing. Check for normal plantar creases and long bone integrity. Assess for normal movement of legs, signs of talipes (check the soles of the feet)	
Genitalia	*Male* Check if penis appears normal and no presence of epispadias Epstein's pearl at tip of penis? Are both testes descended in a normal scrotal sac?	*Female* Normal appearance with labia majora slightly oedematous Any sign of vaginal skin tags or overlarge clitoris?
Spine	Check the integrity of the spine by placing the baby tummy down over the hand whilst the baby is suspended in the air (with large babies let the baby's knees rest on the cot) which allows the vertebrae to open slightly. Gently draw a finger down the spine from the nape of the hair to the coccyx (do not drag the skin). Check for integrity of the spine, presence of hair tufts, sacral dimple and birth marks. Rotate the baby so that you can view and inspect the side of the baby which until now has been facing away from you	
Eyes	Check that both eyes are present and for normal appearance in terms of shape, size and alignment. During the period after birth the baby is often attentive and can demonstrate the ability to 'fixate'	
Skin	Assess the condition of the skin, noting any sign of trauma. Check for rashes and birth marks, noting size, shape and colour as necessary	
Anus	Note appearance and position of anal opening and if the baby passed meconium in utero or soon after delivery. The anus can only be termed as 'patent' if it looks normal and there is evidence of the passage of meconium	
Urine	Passage of urine should be noted and, if witnessed, whether the flow was normal	
Reflexes	These will be assessed when the examination of the newborn is performed, but it should be noticeable if the baby blinks, grasps a finger or if he/she can suckle	

Physical Examination of the Newborn at a Glance, First Edition. Denise (Dee) Campbell and Lyn Dolby.
© 2018 John Wiley & Sons, Ltd. Published 2018 by John Wiley & Sons, Ltd.

The birth of a baby is a significant event in the life of his/her parents. For many mothers, the minutes after birth are full of many emotions, including concern about the baby's condition.

At birth, an immediate concern usually relates to the baby's ability to accomplish the initial changes that are required in order to adapt and survive outside the uterus (see Chapters 8 and 10). However, occasionally an abnormality that was not detected during pregnancy presents at or soon after birth. For example, the baby may exhibit signs of a chromosomal abnormality, heart condition or limb abnormality. At these moments, the level of professional sensitivity, knowledge and understanding employed will make a significant difference to the parents as the initial impact of the issue of concern sinks in. However, it is paramount that if anomalies are found, these concerns must be expressed to the parents followed by an explanation regarding the action that will be taken.

Most of the babies that are examined will have no problem adapting to extrauterine life. Therefore, this is a time for the parents to get to know the signs of a healthy baby and what are issues of concern. Parents also need to be made aware that their baby is undergoing considerable physiological changes and should not be viewed as a 'miniature adult'. The neonatal period denotes the duration of time when most of the major adaptations to extrauterine life take place. This is why the assessment of neonatal health and well-being commences with the initial examination at birth, followed by the examination of the newborn within 72 hours of birth and finally the 6–8 week examination with the GP, unless there is any cause for concern.

Initial examination at birth

Under normal circumstances, this initial examination can be performed within the first hour post birth, after the parents have had time to look at and cuddle their baby. The examination should be performed where it can be easily witnessed by the parents and the lighting is good, particularly in natural daylight. Hands should be washed and dried prior to the examination and everything required should be close at hand (e.g. scales and baby clothes). The examination should be performed quickly and comprehensively, only uncovering the part of the baby to be examined and re-covering the baby as soon as is practicable in order to assist the baby to maintain normal body temperature during a time when this has not yet stabilised.

The initial examination should always include the following points.

• Commence with an exploration of the maternal and neonatal notes, assessing for relevant predisposing factors that may indicate the possibility of compromise to newborn health. Any issue arising during the antenatal period and/or correspondence from the paediatric team or other professional expert or institution should also be taken into account and the parents' knowledge of this ascertained.
• Parent(s) should always be informed about what the examination process entails, their understanding of this assessed and their ability to understand the language used also needs to be determined.
• Parental consent for the examination must always be obtained and the parents made aware that the baby may cry but that this is usually because it has lost the boundaries of the uterus around it and because of the stimuli of light, touch and sound.

• Parent(s) should be asked for their impression of their baby's health and if they have any concerns and these may also include issues that have arisen during the antenatal period.
• The baby should be examined in full view of the parents, or a parent if circumstances surrounding birth preclude this from happening.
• The examination should follow a systematic process in order not to miss any part of the examination (Table 19.1).
• The parent(s) should be fully informed of the findings of the examination and be made aware of their baby's abilities even at this young age, for example, the ability to fixate with the eyes and the neurological reflexes that are present and why.
• Specific newborn care practices should be discussed if they relate to the findings of the examination or culture and/or religion. For example, the parents may come from a culture that frequently 'swaddles' their babies, or it is common in the parents' religion or culture to circumcise baby boys but an epispadias has been noted on examination (see Genitalia in Table 19.1).

Post examination

Any anomaly must be appropriately and accurately recorded and referral sought if required. In the event of birth marks it is particularly important to draw a body diagram to depict position, colour and size, especially if the birth mark could be confused with non-accidental injury (see Chapters 30 and 31).

If not already accomplished, the baby should be weighed naked. Attention should be paid at this stage to making sure that the scales are properly calibrated, that the examiner does not accidently lean on the scales or that part of the scale is touching anything else that may cause an inaccurate reading to be taken.

Administration of vitamin K should already have been discussed with the parents, but this should be broached again. The choice of method of administration depends in part on the routes of administration available in differing parts of the country. The parents need to be clear what vitamin K is administered for, where and how it is administered, and what needs to occur in the future if oral vitamin K is used.

Finally, the baby should be dressed and a hat put on his/her head. There may still be some residual dampness within the hair and a hat assists in keeping the baby warm whilst his/her temperature control mechanisms stabilise. The hat should be removed after approximately 6 hours in the healthy term baby, as he/she should be able to maintain his//her own temperature reasonably well by this time.

The examiner must portray good role model behaviour from the start. For example, if placing the baby in the cot, he/she should be placed on his/her back, with the bed clothing placed appropriately to assist in safe sleeping practices (see Chapter 5).

Returning the baby to the parents may only necessitate placing a nappy on the baby if the mother wishes to hold her baby skin-to-skin. This position will reduce stress on the baby, settling and calming the baby's vital signs and encourages the baby to root and breastfeed. This is a period of time for the parents to be left to bond, to hydrate and have some light refreshment whilst the examination is documented.

All documentation should be fully completed, including any discussions with the paediatrician if required, the weight of the baby, any parental concerns and their wishes regarding method of infant feeding. If vitamin K has been administered, parental consent, the dose, batch number and how/where given should be clearly recorded.

20 Daily examination of the newborn – overview

Table 20.1 Main issues covered in the daily examination of the newborn.

Aspect	Observe and assess the following elements	
Colour	Pink/well perfused Jaundiced: predisposing factors, does the baby appear well?	
Head	Status of moulding, bruising or other trauma arising from delivery Only measure the head circumference if there is any query concerning the measurement taken at birth or any other factors that can impact on head size	
Neck	Observe for signs of chafing, soreness, etc.	
Palate	Only review state of palate if there are signs of concern (e.g. milk often comes out of the baby's nose)	
Posture/behaviour	Assess tone, good flexion, normal movements and responsiveness to speech, light and touch	
Heart rate	Apex beat should still reflect normality (100–160/min), but only reassess if there are signs of concern	
Respiratory	Respiratory rate should still reflect normality (30–60/min), but only reassess if there are signs of concern	
Temperature	Temperature should be within the realms of normality (36.8–37.5°C). Unless the baby has previously been noted to be cold or feels cooler than expected to the touch (chest and between scapulae), there should be no need to take the baby's temperature	
Umbilicus	Depending on the number of days since birth, check if clamp secure, no signs of flaring or odour and that normal process of separation is occurring	
Upper limbs	Assess that general movement is within the range of normality	
Lower limbs	Assess that general movement is within the range of normality	
Genitalia/excretion	*Male* Assess for signs of soreness or infection, bruising or condition of hydrocele if present Is there a good urine flow on micturition?	*Female* Assess for signs of soreness or infection Signs or mucous, pseudomenstruation?
	Note if the baby has passed urine or meconium and how often – link to feeding ability Is the anus patent? The passage of nitrates may be seen as a small orange patch in the nappy Any sign of nappy rash?	
Eyes	Assess if eyes are 'sticky' or if there are signs of infection Assess alertness and responsiveness	
Skin – general	Assess the condition of the skin, noting any sign of trauma. Check for rashes and birth marks, noting size, shape and colour as necessary	
Reflexes	Reflexes will be assessed when the examination of the newborn is performed, but the ability of the baby to blink, grasp a finger and suckle should be observed Any odd or abnormal movements should be observed, documented (including any related findings) and a referral made to the paediatric team	
Maternal health and well-being	Maternal–parental interactions with their newborn baby should be noticed in a sensitive manner Maternal fears or concerns should be listened to and not quickly dismissed Time spent with a mother is never 'time wasted'	

The first 3–4 weeks after a baby's birth constitutes a significant period of learning not only for the parents, but also the baby. Most babies have managed to accomplish the initial adaptations to extrauterine life, but their continuing progress and development will need careful observation during the neonatal period. It is for this reason that the daily examination is an important part of neonatal care, as it is not only a time of observation and reassessment of the baby's progress, but also a time of sharing information with the parents in relation to their baby's physiological status and his/her ability to interact with and react to the people and the world around him/her. This is also a time when parents should be reminded that their baby is not a miniature adult, but that he/she is undergoing considerable physiological changes.

Daily examination of the newborn

Under normal circumstances, this daily examination should be performed when it is convenient for both mother and baby. Preferably, the baby should be in the 'quiet, alert' state of consciousness if their ongoing development of health and well-being is to be comprehensively assessed.

As with the initial examination, the baby should be examined where he/she can be easily witnessed by the parents and the lighting is good, preferably in natural daylight. Hands should be washed and dried prior to the examination and everything required should be close at hand (e.g. clean nappy, bowl of warm water for cleaning purposes).

Always assess the baby's temperature first, particularly if this is the first daily examination or if the parents have voiced concerns about their baby's behaviour. If the baby is over 6 hours old and still has a hat on indoors, this can be removed and the parents informed that babies only need hats if outdoors (warm hat for cold conditions and sunhat at other times). If the baby has previously been noted to have had a low temperature, use a suitable means of temperature measurement so that an accurate assessment can be made. If the baby's temperature is below normal thresholds, then the baby should not be undressed (unless skin-to-skin is advocated) and a hat should be placed on the baby's head. An investigation should be commenced to determine why the baby became cold and appropriate management undertaken.

The daily examination should always include the following points.

• Commence with an exploration of the maternal and neonatal notes in order to determine if any changes have occurred since birth. If the examiner is seeing this baby for the first time, he/she should check for relevant predisposing factors that may indicate the possibility of compromise to newborn health. Any issue arising during the antenatal period and/or correspondence from the paediatric team or other professional expert or institution should also be taken into account and the parents' knowledge of this ascertained.
• Discussion with the parent(s) in relation to any concerns that they may have and, as with the initial examination, they should always be informed about what the examination process entails, their understanding of this assessed and their ability to understand the language used also needs to be determined.
• Parental consent for the examination must always be obtained.
• The baby should be examined in full view of the parent(s).
• The examination should follow a systematic process in order not to miss any part of the examination (Table 20.1).
• The parent(s) should be fully informed of the findings of the examination.
• If appropriate, they should be gently informed about physiological and pathological jaundice, particularly if the baby has obvious signs of trauma or bruising from delivery.

• The progression of feeding should be discussed and it should be ascertained if the mother requires extra help or if the baby needs to be observed when feeding.
• Skin care and care of the umbilicus is important as many parents are unaware of how thin the baby's skin layer is, or how any preparation used on the skin can be partly absorbed. However, they need to be aware of how detrimental urine and faeces can be to the skin and how to avoid soreness and chafing. They also need to be informed of the skin preparations that can be used (if really necessary) that have little impact on the physiology of the skin. The practitioner needs to be fully conversant about the contemporary literature that is available in order to accomplish this effectively.
• This is a good time to discuss the baby's abilities, or to point out signs of good health, such as how alert the baby is, its attentiveness, pointing out how well perfused the baby is through its colour, how to check the baby is warm enough (place back of hand on the baby's chest or between the scapulae) or demonstrating that the baby has normal muscle tone.
• As with the initial examination, specific newborn care practices should be discussed. It may only be during the daily examination that particular care practices relating to culture and/or religion come to light. For example, the parents may come from a culture that frequently 'swaddles' their babies.

Post examination

Any anomaly must be appropriately and accurately recorded and referral sought if required. In the event of skin changes, it should be determined if these are caused by normal physiology, such as the often apparent erythema toxicum neonatorum, or if they are of a nature that is more concerning such as an odd subtle birthmark or the presence of pustular spots that may be indicative of infection.

If the baby was found to have been placed on his/her side or stomach to sleep, the practitioner needs to discuss the salient aspects of safer sleeping in a sensitive but informed manner (see Chapter 5). This may also mean that the sleeping position of the baby in the cot is demonstrated so that the parents not only have an audio image, but also a visual one.

A comprehensive record of the examination must be completed, including an indication of how feeding is progressing and the quantity of 'wet' and 'dirty' nappies (and if the consistency is changing). Any parental concerns should be recorded and information given in response and/or actions taken.

Maternal well-being

The daily examination is not just about reviewing the baby's health and well-being, it is also a time when maternal or parental reactions to their newborn baby can be quietly observed. The 'bonding' process between mother and baby is not always an easy one and not all mothers love their child the instant they are born. For some, these early days are a period of change, uncertainty and concern about their own abilities as parents. For others, there may be other issues that are impacting on their ability to care for themselves, let alone this newborn baby. The effect of the mother's mental health on herself, the baby and her family can be considerable (Royal College of Midwives, 2014; RCOG, 2017; Swingler et al., 2017).

The daily examination may at first appear to be solely focused on the baby but observing the interaction between baby and parents is just as important in relation to health and well-being. Practitioners should be conversant with the available guidance and policies and need to be aware of any shortcomings within their own knowledge base if early recognition of those women who need extra assistance if they are to be provided with appropriate care. Remember, the time you spend with a mother is never 'time wasted'.

Newborn blood spot screening

Table 21.1 The conditions that are part of the newborn blood spot (NBS) screening programme.

Condition	Details	Management
Sickle cell disease (SCD)	Part of the NBS screening programme in England since 2006 An autosomal recessive inherited condition that affects haemoglobin Incidence: 1 in 2200 babies in England 1 in 74 carriers are detected Present at birth, but signs of SCD may not appear until after 4 months of age Babies with this condition will need specialist care throughout their lives If untreated: high risk of death or complications from treatable infections, severe acute anaemia and stroke in the first few years of life It can cause attacks of very severe pain, life-threatening infections and anaemia Ongoing parental support is required	Early treatment recommended, including childhood immunisations Oral penicillin and Prevenar vaccine before 3 months of age to reduce the chance of serious illness Note: babies with beta thalassaemia major – the most serious form of thalassaemia – will generally be detected by screening, but carriers are not detected
Cystic fibrosis	Part of the NBS screening programme in England since 2007 An autosomal recessive inherited condition affecting the digestive system and lungs Incidence: 1 in 2500 in the UK Symptoms usually begin in early childhood, with poor weight gain and frequent chest infections If untreated: leads to lung damage, poor growth and development Survival: mean age = 41	Early treatment – high-energy diet, medication and regular physiotherapy commencing by 30 days of age Note: some babies require a second blood sample for further testing on day 21 Not all carriers will be identified
Congenital hypothyroidism	Part of the NBS screening programme in England since 1981 There are a number of causes for hypothyroidism, but it is not usually inherited Incidence: 1 in 3000 babies in the UK A condition in which insufficient thyroxine is produced Babies do not have any problems at birth, but if left untreated permanent physical and mental disability will develop	Treatment commences with thyroxine therapy by 21 days of age to allow normal development

Table 21.2 Inherited metabolic diseases (IMDs) that are part of the NBS screening programme.

The following six IMDs are all autosomal recessive inherited metabolic diseases, which cause the following problems:	
Phenylketonuria (PKU) Screened by blood spot since early 1970s	Causes: difficulty with breaking down the phenylalanine amino acid Incidence: 1 in 10 000 in the UK
Medium-chain acyl-CoA dehydrogenase deficiency (MCADD) Screened since 2007–2008	Causes: a difficulty with breaking down fat Incidence: 1 in 10 000 in the UK
Maple syrup urine disease (MSUD) Included in screening since 2015	Causes: difficulty with breaking down leucine, isoleucine and valine amino acids Incidence: 1 in 116 000 in the UK
Isovaleric acidaemia (IVA) Included in screening since 2015	Causes: difficulty with breaking down the leucine amino acid Incidence: 1 in 155 000 in the EU
Glutaric aciduria type 1 (GA1) Included in screening since 2015	Causes: difficulty with breaking down lysine and tryptophan amino acids Incidence: 1 in 110 000 in the EU
Homocysteinuria (pyridoxine unresponsive) (HCU) Included in screening since 2015	Prevents the breakdown of the homocysteine amino acid Incidence: 1 in 144 000 in UK

For further detail on the six IMDs go to: https://www.gov.uk/government/uploads/system/uploads/attachment_data/file/511688/Guidelines_for_Newborn_Blood_Spot_Sampling_January_2016.pdf

Physical Examination of the Newborn at a Glance, First Edition. Denise (Dee) Campbell and Lyn Dolby.
© 2018 John Wiley & Sons, Ltd. Published 2018 by John Wiley & Sons, Ltd.

NHS newborn blood spot screening programme

The UK National Screening Committee issues guidance, support and training on various conditions that can affect the health of individuals. For some conditions, a national programme of screening has been established in order to detect these conditions early, provide pre-emptive treatment and reduce the cost to the health of the individual as well as the financial costs incurred for later recognition and treatment. Therefore, as with any widespread screening programme, the cost of screening has to be balanced with the acceptability of the screening rationale and method by individuals, the impact on the health of the individual, the prevalence of the condition and the ability to treat or manage the condition effectively.

Newborn blood spot (NBS) screening is one of the areas that is covered by a national screening programme. It enables identification of babies who may have rare but serious conditions. The number of babies affected may be small, but early detection, referral and treatment can help to improve their health and prevent severe disability or, in some cases, death.

The UK National Screening Committee recommends that all babies are offered screening and at present this consists of the following:

- Three conditions as shown in Table 21.1
  1 Sickle cell disease (SCD);
  2 Cystic fibrosis (CF);
  3 Congenital hypothyroidism (CHT).
- And six inherited metabolic diseases (IMDs; Table 21.2):
  1 Phenylketonuria (PKU);
  2 Medium-chain acyl-CoA dehydrogenase deficiency (MCADD);
  3 Maple syrup urine disease (MSUD);
  4 Isovaleric acidaemia (IVA);
  5 Glutaric aciduria type 1 (GA1);
  6 Homocysteinuria (pyridoxine unresponsive) (HCU).

Prior to or during the antenatal booking session, a copy of the booklet, 'Screening tests for you and your baby', should be given to all women. This is also a good time to ascertain from the parents if there is a family history of any of the IMDs so that early screening can be offered if appropriate. For women whose first language is not English, translated versions of the information booklet are available (www.gov.uk/government/publications/screening-tests-for-you-and-your-baby-description-in-brief).

It is important to offer NBS screening to all parents and to check that those who have just moved into the area with a newborn baby have not missed out on the opportunity to have their baby screened. As with any procedure, parents need comprehensive information about the screening programme, what it tests for and the possible outcomes if their baby tests positive for any of the conditions and how the sampling is conducted.

As NBS screening usually takes place on day 5 post birth (day of birth = day 0), NBS screening should ideally be discussed again at least 24 hours prior to the procedure. This gives parents the opportunity to think about the information that they have been given, view the details on the Public Health England, National Screening Committee website and decide whether they wish to give their consent. When verbal consent to NBS screening has been given, it should be clearly recorded as 'consent given' in the NHS Trust maternal/neonatal record and/or electronic record and the Personal Child Health Record.

Parental consent to any research linked to the NBS screening programme should also be ascertained and they should be informed that they can find further information via the website (www.nhs.uk/Conditions/pregnancy-and-baby/Pages/newborn-blood-spot-cards.aspx). If a parent does not wish to be contacted about future research in relation to their baby's sample, they will need to know and see evidence that the words 'No research contact' have been recorded clearly on the blood spot card. However, parents do need to know that patient identifiable information may be stored by the NHS Sickle Cell and Thalassaemia Screening Programme. The information relating to this is available online (www.gov.uk/newborn-outcomes-project-definition-and-implementation).

Parents can also decline screening for one or more of the first three conditions (SCD, CF and CHT), but the six IMDs can only be declined as a group. In this instance, a clear record should be made in the NHS Trust maternal/neonatal record and/or electronic record and the Personal Child Health Record. It must state clearly which test is being declined and if possible the rationale for the parents decision. When NBS screening is declined for only one or some of the conditions, the blood spot card should be completed and marked 'Decline – XX' (where XX is the condition(s) that has been declined) and add the rationale if given.

In the event that consent is declined for NBS screening per se, the records should clearly state this decision and rationale if possible. The blood spot card should also be completed but this time it should be marked 'Decline – all conditions' and rationale given if available prior to being sent to the laboratory. Local procedures should be followed in relation to informing the Child Health Records Department, the GP, health visitor and the NBS lead midwife/manager. A separate letter will also be sent to the parents, but they should also be informed verbally who they can contact if they change their minds or would like to discuss any aspect of the screening process or require further information. All of this will need to be recorded in the Personal Child Health Record.

The sampling process

For the purpose of NBS screening, the day of birth is counted as 'day 0'. The blood spot sample should be taken on day 5 for all babies, but in exceptional circumstances the sample may be taken between days 5 and 8 or may need to be repeated. For example, the baby may have been born prematurely or has recently had a blood transfusion which can affect the test results.

NHS Public Health England produced 'Guidelines for Newborn Blood Spot Sampling' in 2016. This document sets out the information about the rationale for screening, parental information and consent, the sampling procedure and the issues that lead to repeat tests because of poor or inadequate samples or false positive or negative results. They also provide an e-learning, visual training module to enable healthcare professionals achieve the best possible sample and understand the implications of poor practices. All healthcare professionals are strongly advised to access the guidelines and the e-learning resource (https://cpdscreening.phe.org.uk/elearning) at regular intervals in order to maintain contemporary knowledge about the programme and the rationale for the tests currently offered. However, local guidelines and procedures must also follow where necessary in addition to the guidelines.

22 Hearing screening

Figure 22.1 Automated Otto Acoustic Emissions (AOAE) testing.
Source: http://kasper-achs-block3.wikispaces.com/file/view/hearing_test.jpg/235297155/230x152/hearing_test.jpg Accessed June 2017. Licensed under CC BY-SA 3.0.

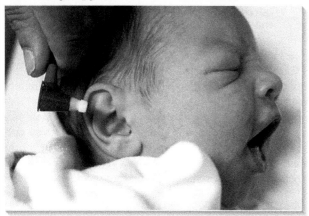

Figure 22.2 Automated Auditory Brainstem Response (AABR) testing.
Source: http://farm3.staticflickr.com/2341/2130329339_a737b3867e _z.jpg
Accessed June 2017. Reproduced with permission of Thomas Widmann.

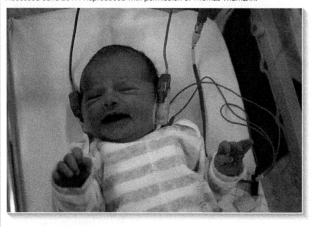

Figure 22.3 AABR testing.
Source: http://farm1.staticflickr.com/49/174964974
_dd44db3940_z.jpg
Accessed June 2017. Reproduced with permission of Dean Johnson.

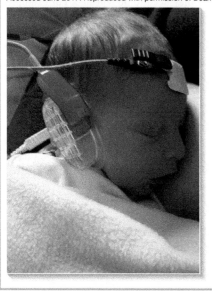

Figure 22.4 AABR testing.
Source: https://www.flickr.com/photos/jacob-davies/with/4030589130
Accessed June 2017. Reproduced with permission of Jacob Davies.

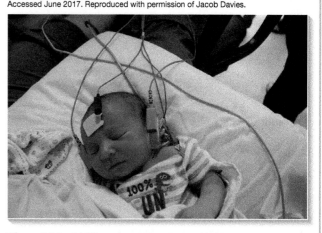

Figure 22.5 AABR testing.
Source: https://www.flickr.com/photos/zepplinrace/10506904914
Accessed June 2017. Reproduced with permission of Matthew Sheales.

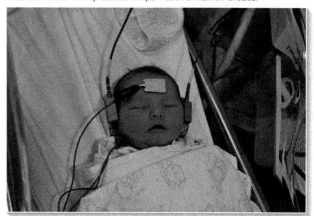

Physical Examination of the Newborn at a Glance, First Edition. Denise (Dee) Campbell and Lyn Dolby.
© 2018 John Wiley & Sons, Ltd. Published 2018 by John Wiley & Sons, Ltd.

Early screening for full or partial deafness reduces many long-term health issues and the associated health costs. Detection of a problem with appropriate management improves intellectual, social, psychological and communication outcomes.

Informed choice

Leaflets are available in several languages and discussions with healthcare professionals can clarify any concerns. Information should be shared about:

- Procedures involved in screening;
- Painless nature of the various tests involved;
- Follow-up processes that may be required;
- Advantages of early detection;
- Only known risk – the possibility of a false positive and the associated anxieties involved;
- Why false positives occur: for example, uncooperative, distressed newborn; background noise or interference; faulty equipment; or temporary deafness and blocking of the auditory canal.

Referral for screening

Most commonly, screening takes place on the postnatal ward prior to discharge and within 48 hours of birth. It is performed by trained audiologists who make daily visits to the ward. In some circumstances, such as following a home birth or over a bank holiday, referral may be required to an alternative designated professional for the tests. This may be to an individual (such as a health visitor) or to an audiology clinic. This should ideally be within a month of birth for a healthy term newborn but can be still carried out up to 3 months after delivery. For a premature infant, the optimum time is calculated based on the expected date of delivery.

Explaining the screening tests

There are two screening tests available for routine use at birth.

Automated Otto Acoustic Emissions (AOAE)

This can be used from a few hours after birth. It is painless and takes only a few minutes (Figure 22.1). The parent/carer can stay with the newborn throughout. A soft earpiece is inserted into the ear and clicking noises are played through it. A normal cochlea will then emit a responsive reaction, detected by the test equipment. A clear response from both ears is reassuring of no early onset deafness. This test has the advantage of its non-invasive speedy result but is associated with higher false negative rates. In the absence of a clear response, the second screening test is then used.

Automated Auditory Brainstem Response (AABR)

This test requires a restful, preferably sleeping, newborn and a suitably quiet environment away from other noisy stimuli (Figures 22.2, 22.3, 22.4 and 22.5). Parents or carers can stay with the newborn and can be reassured that the test is painless and takes only 5–15 minutes. This test examines the full pathway for hearing, going beyond the cochlea to monitor brainstem responses. The test involves sounds being played through head phones or occasionally ear probes may be used. Sensors are typically attached on the baby's forehead and shoulder but sometimes also on the nape of the neck. Before the sensors are put in place the skin should be cleaned with special wipes and allowed to dry, then a conductive gel is applied and the sensors attached with sticky pads.

Professional responsibilities

The professional carrying out the physical examination of the newborn must verify that one of the following has occurred.

Screening has been discussed but consent was withheld

- A non-judgemental approach is taken and everything documented.
- GP and health visitor are made aware.
- The parent/carer has been encouraged to monitor ongoing progress using the developmental checklists and notify any concerns.

Screening has been completed with a clear response in both ears

- Everything has been appropriately documented.
- Possibility of late onset deafness is discussed and the parent/carer has been encouraged to monitor ongoing progress using the developmental checklists and notify any concerns.
- A clear response letter has been given to the parent/carer.
- Risk factors and follow-up needs have been considered.

Screening has been completed with an inconclusive or non-clear response in one or both ears

- Everything has been appropriately documented.
- A follow-up hearing specialist or audiology clinic appointment has been arranged for 4 weeks after the initial tests.
- The carer has been given an explanation and been encouraged to monitor their newborn's progress using the developmental checklists.

Risk factors (Sutton et al., 2012)

Prior to the routine early neonatal screening programmes, only those considered at high risk were screened and as many as 50% of those with full or partial deafness were missed. The problems were often not identified until they became clinically apparent. The presence of risk factors for both early and late onset deafness still has an important role in decision making but this is now in addition to routine screening. Even when the AABR screening test is clear from both ears, the presence of risk factors requires a referral for audiological and behavioural assessment at 7–9 months.

Risk factors include:

- Congenital rubella, cytomegalovirus or toxoplasmosis;
- Parents concerned about a family history even after clear screening;
- A newborn with a syndrome associated with deafness (e.g. Down's syndrome);
- Cranium or facial abnormalities (including cleft palate);
- Parental or professional concerns related to development;
- Temporal bone fracture;
- Severe unconjugated hyperbilirubinaemia.

Additionally, there are risk factors so likely to affect partial or full hearing loss that a **full audiological referral** should routinely be made for when the newborn is 4 weeks old:

- Atresia of the external meatus;
- Microtia (under-developed pinna);
- Bacterial meningitis;
- Meningococcal septicaemia.

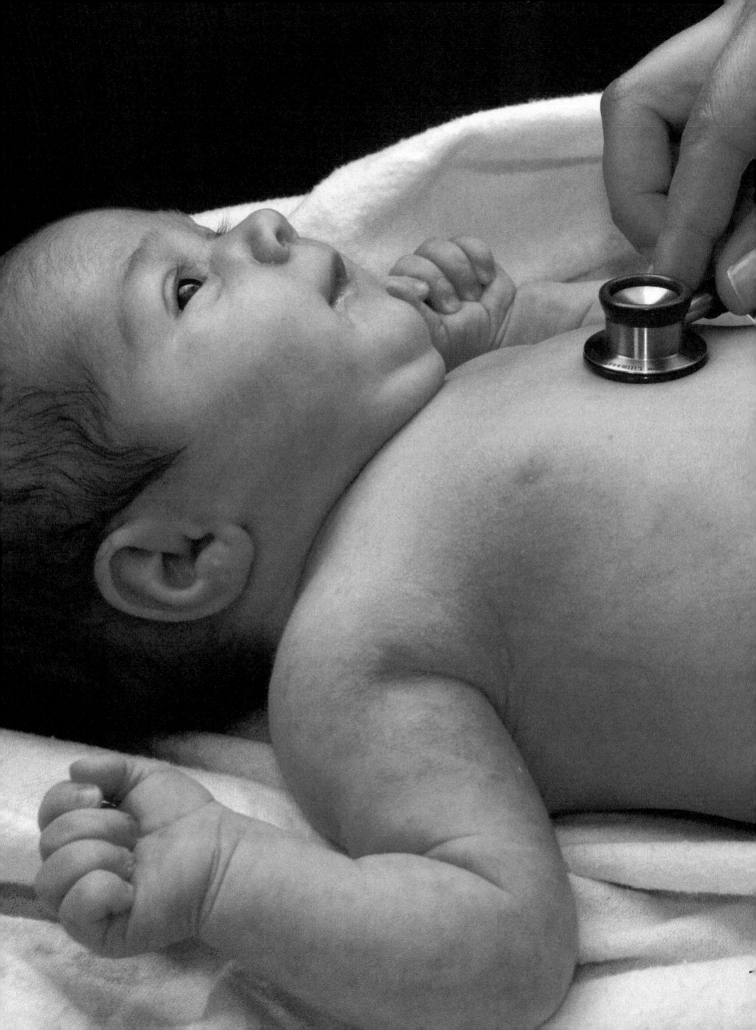

Prior to the physical examination

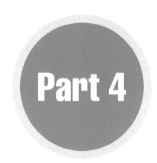

Part 4

Chapters

23 Preparing to examine

Figure 23.1 Neonatal stethoscope head (chest piece).

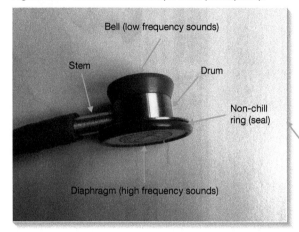

Bell (low frequency sounds)

Stem

Drum

Non-chill
ring (seal)

Diaphragm (high frequency sounds)

Figure 23.2 Neonatal stethoscope.

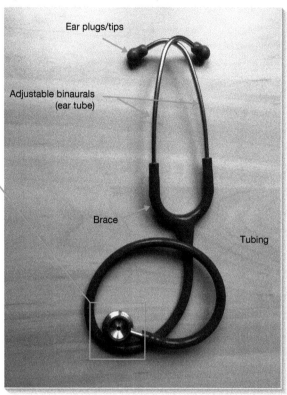

Ear plugs/tips

Adjustable binaurals
(ear tube)

Brace

Tubing

Figure 23.3 Pocket ophthalmoscope with the practitioners side facing uppermost.

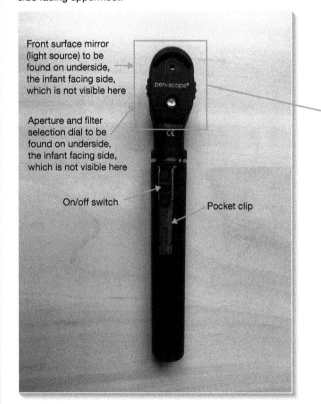

Front surface mirror
(light source) to be
found on underside,
the infant facing side,
which is not visible here

Aperture and filter
selection dial to be
found on underside,
the infant facing side,
which is not visible here

On/off switch

Pocket clip

Figure 23.4 Ophthalmoscope head – practitioner side.

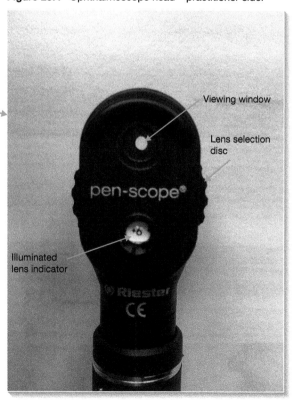

Viewing window

Lens selection
disc

Illuminated
lens indicator

Physical Examination of the Newborn at a Glance, First Edition. Denise (Dee) Campbell and Lyn Dolby.
© 2018 John Wiley & Sons, Ltd. Published 2018 by John Wiley & Sons, Ltd.

Information gathering

The physical examination commences with the review of all relevant histories, to inform the examination and its outcome. All information gleaned from the records should be viewed as a screening tool that informs the practitioner about the infant's higher or lower probability of risk. Whilst it is possible that the competent practitioner would identify any physical abnormalities even without this additional information, this knowledge enables an individualised approach towards risk and greater sensitivity to the specific concerns of the family. History alone can alert the practitioner to further screening and diagnostic care required (aligned to local policies and protocols) and any child protection issues. Furthermore, a combination of prior history and the current examination will guide additional screening and referrals – including to whom, when, where and how these referrals should be made.

Awareness of a client's history is a part of the professional's role. This must be treated with sensitivity on a 'need to know' basis to support client confidentiality. Analysis of the information is from the perspective of how aspects may directly, or indirectly, impact on the current health and future development of the infant.

Predicting concerns

Specific screening tests will already have been performed antenatally and the results will impact on the neonatal examination. This is not only linked to occasions when screening has identified a higher risk situation, but also because the discussions around reliability of screening tests will have introduced awareness for the family around false positive and false negative results. Sadly, they may have been left with increased awareness of neonatal health risks but without a complete guarantee that their baby is not affected. Diagnostic tests may also have been carried out or may have been decided against because of their own inherent health risks for the fetus. The practitioner is expected to have some knowledge around how genetic and inherent conditions or physical abnormalities occur to enable informed discussion. The practitioner may wish to seek advice and increase awareness about these before approaching the family. Updates from the midwife providing daily care ensures the most up-to-date information.

Parents may consider the physical examination as a way they can be reassured about the health of their baby. The practitioner should be aware of tests that have been carried out and their results before entering a conversation with the family. It is essential that the limitations of the examination are clearly explained. Reassurances may follow the examination and greater clarity may be possible around identified concerns but the examination is itself only a screening tool with its own limitations. Fetal transition to newborn life is still ongoing at 72 hours so the examination can only relate to the specific moment in time that it takes place and this is particularly true for the heart.

Collecting equipment

- **Tape measure** – disposable, flexible, clearly printed in centimetres and non-stretchable.
- **Stethoscope** (Figures 23.1 and 23.2) – a specific paediatric one (some adult-sized cardiac stethoscopes can be fitted with a paediatric use diaphragm). The stethoscope must be clean and maintained in good working order with no signs of damage related to the diaphragm, ear pieces or tubing; dual head able to rotate 180° without resistance; and working seals to prevent air loss (air escape noises can impact on hearing heart sounds and murmurs).
- **Ophthalmoscope** (Figures 23.3 and 23.4) – a direct vision one. The ophthalmoscope required for viewing the red reflex can be a basic design but must be clean and maintained in good working order providing a good light source, large round aperture and means to focus the reflected image.
- **Documentation** – the notes should have already been reviewed for risk factors but the examiner will need the paediatric and postnatal aspects to record the results. The Personal Child Health Record (PCHR), also known as the 'Red book', is provided for every newborn baby to maintain an ongoing health and development record. This includes a page for the neonatal physical examination results.
- **Clean nappy and changing equipment** – to be used as required to facilitate clear viewing of the genitalia, buttocks and upper thigh and also to enable accurate examination for femoral pulses and developmental dysplasia of the hips (DDH).

Considering the environment

The environment for the examination can affect the neonate, family and practitioner as well as impacting on the ability to communicate.

- **Privacy** – away from the hearing of others to allow opportunity for honest and sensitive communications.
- **Warmth** – the infant is undressed and is either uncovered or semicovered during the examination so a warm room is needed to help the balance of the baby's immature thermoregulation system. An item of clothing or a blanket should be available to cover areas of the baby that have already been fully visualised and examined or between elements of the examination (perhaps when communicating with the mother).
- **Lighting** – this must provide the opportunity to see the infant's skin colour in good natural lighting. Additionally, the opportunity to reduce lighting can help calm an infant and enable the red reflex examination.
- **Infant position** – safe, on a firm mattress and at a suitable height for good access by the practitioner.
- **Access to handwashing facilities** – Handwashing is required before and after the examination. It must occur after any nappy changing procedure or contact with vomit, urine or stool. This is a standard precaution within infection control.

Some practitioners perform the examination on a resuscitaire within a nursery. This can be an appropriate environment with parental consent but may require reassurances around the equipment present. It also requires comfortable seating for the parents who should not be excluded.

24 Infection control

Figure 24.1 The stages of handwashing or gel application.
Source: WHO (2009).

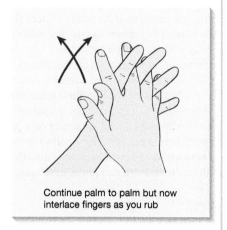

Wet hands and apply soap or
apply hand gel to dry hands

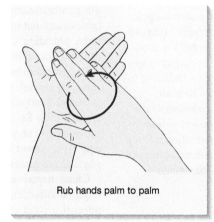

Rub hands palm to palm

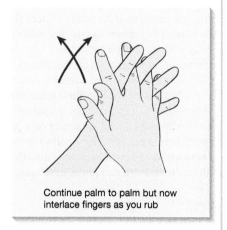

Continue palm to palm but now
interlace fingers as you rub

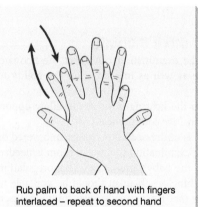

Rub palm to back of hand with fingers
interlaced – repeat to second hand

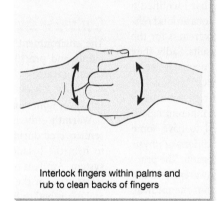

Interlock fingers within palms and
rub to clean backs of fingers

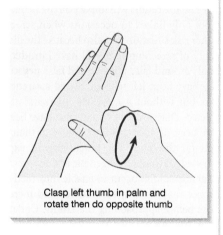

Clasp left thumb in palm and
rotate then do opposite thumb

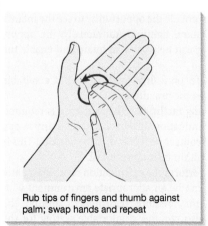

Rub tips of fingers and thumb against
palm; swap hands and repeat

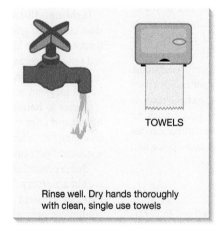

TOWELS

Rinse well. Dry hands thoroughly
with clean, single use towels

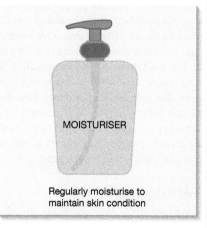

MOISTURISER

Regularly moisturise to
maintain skin condition

Physical Examination of the Newborn at a Glance, First Edition. Denise (Dee) Campbell and Lyn Dolby.
© 2018 John Wiley & Sons, Ltd. Published 2018 by John Wiley & Sons, Ltd.

This chapter considers the infection control responsibilities of the professional performing the physical examination. They must:

- Ensure that they do not introduce infection;
- Identify infection already affecting the infant;
- Initiate appropriate treatment of any infection;
- Control against spread of infection;
- Participate in the education of parents;
- Lead by example.

Infection risks

The risk of healthcare-associated infections during a hospital stay is 5–15% within developed countries, rising to as high as 19% in developing countries and increasing further for higher risk infants born prematurely or admitted to intensive care facilities (World Health Organization, 2009). A number of factors increase infection risks for the newborn:

- Increased levels of bacteria within hospital environments – airborne as well as carried by staff and equipment;
- Lowered resistance when newborn;
- Exposure as a fetus (e.g. via prolonged rupture of membranes);
- Increased maternal infection risk (e.g. because of anaemia or operative delivery), for example;
- Close proximity within maternity wards increasing risk of spread;
- Sharing of equipment (see Chapter 23);
- Warm atmosphere allowing bacteria to multiply;
- High visitor numbers;
- Increased likelihood of body fluid exposure.

Infection prevention

Infection prevention is enhanced through an understanding of how infection may be transmitted during the physical examination and the standard precautions that reduce this occurrence. The value of decontamination during hand hygiene was first appreciated by Ignaz Semmelweis in 1847. He was investigating considerably higher levels of puerperal fever in the clinic visited by medical students compared with one run solely by midwives. His breakthrough came when a colleague was accidentally cut by a medical student's scalpel during a post mortem and died displaying the symptoms of puerperal fever. Semmelweis realised that medical students were carrying infective body particles from the post mortem (despite handwashing). He escalated handwashing to include chlorinated lime, with an immediate 90% reduction in mortality rates. Sadly, his criticism of the medical profession's hygiene and inability to evidence his theories lost him his career (and in time his mental health too). Louis Pasteur later provided the evidence for all that Semmelweis had described and called it antisepsis – providing his own detailed theories around germs and disease.

Hand decontamination

Two categories of bacteria commonly exist on the hands: resident and transient (WHO, 2009). Transient bacteria are more likely to be responsible for cross-infection but are also more responsive to hand hygiene (WHO, 2009). The WHO (2009) 'Guidelines on Hand Hygiene in Health Care' suggest that each mother and baby should be treated as a single patient zone and advocate five points at which hand hygiene is required. These are listed with examples of how they should be applied during the physical examination:

1 **Before patient contact** – on entering the room, before touching the newborn.

2 **Before aseptic tasks** – unlikely to be an element of the physical examination unless a new point of infection is observed that now requires dressing (e.g. omphalitis).

3 **After body fluid exposure risk** – may be obvious from dribbling, posset, vomit, sneeze, nappy change, blood or any exudate, but also occurs when dressing or undressing the newborn, examining the mouth digitally, assessing femoral pulses or developmental dysplasia of the hips, and examination of the groin, genitalia or anus.

4 **After patient contact** – following completion of the physical examination.

5 **After contact with patient surroundings** – on leaving the room, hand gel should be applied outside the door before moving on to the next task. In any situation of source isolation nursing or known infection risk, the hands should be fully rewashed when leaving the room.

Hand decontamination

Handwashing and alcohol gel, hand rub application techniques are illustrated in Figure 24.1. A gel hand rub should only be used if the hands are clean. For the routine procedure involved in the physical examination, gloves are not required, but this should be reconsidered on an individual basis for any additional potential risk, in which case a plastic apron should also be worn to protect clothing.

Hand care

Hands should be examined daily for signs of broken skin, inflammation or torn cuticles (NICE, 2012b). Moisturising prevents drying and cracking from frequent handwashing and alcohol gel use. Nails must be short, smoothly filed and free from nail varnish, extensions or additions. A flat ring band does not prevent good hand hygiene but clothing below the elbow and all other jewellery (including watches) can contaminate and interfere with washing and should be removed (Hautemaniere et al., 2010).

Signs of infection

Early identification enables appropriate management for the health of the infant and prevention of spread. The history and risk factors act as indicators and the signs include:

- Sleepiness with poor feeding;
- Inflammation, redness or an area of localised heat;
- Localised serous fluid or a purulent exudate;
- Vomiting and/or diarrhoea;
- Systemic temperature raised (above 38°C), low (below 36.6°C) or, unstable;
- Increased or reduced respirations or respiratory distress;
- Jitteriness or seizures;
- An area of swelling and/or tenderness;
- Bradycardia;
- Jaundice;
- Apnoea or shock;
- Blood-stained urine (non-pseudomenstruation or urates).

25 Relevant history and risk factors

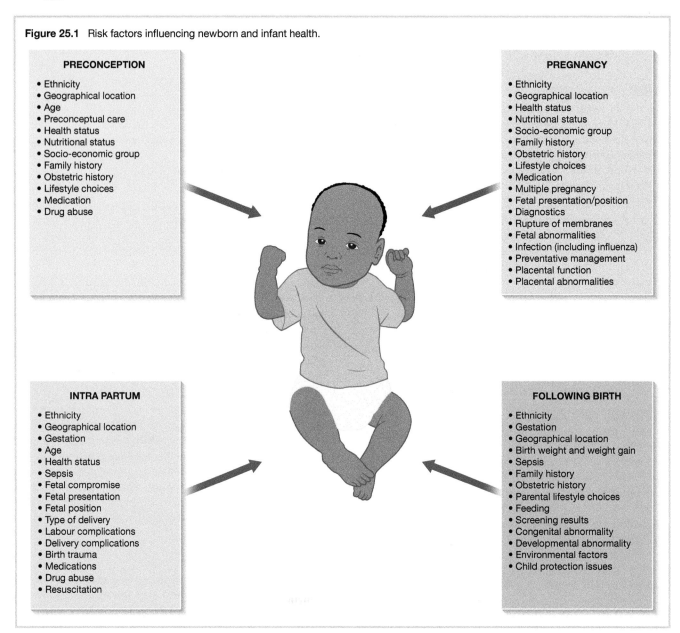

Figure 25.1 Risk factors influencing newborn and infant health.

PRECONCEPTION
- Ethnicity
- Geographical location
- Age
- Preconceptual care
- Health status
- Nutritional status
- Socio-economic group
- Family history
- Obstetric history
- Lifestyle choices
- Medication
- Drug abuse

PREGNANCY
- Ethnicity
- Geographical location
- Health status
- Nutritional status
- Socio-economic group
- Family history
- Obstetric history
- Lifestyle choices
- Medication
- Multiple pregnancy
- Fetal presentation/position
- Diagnostics
- Rupture of membranes
- Fetal abnormalities
- Infection (including influenza)
- Preventative management
- Placental function
- Placental abnormalities

INTRA PARTUM
- Ethnicity
- Geographical location
- Gestation
- Age
- Health status
- Sepsis
- Fetal compromise
- Fetal presentation
- Fetal position
- Type of delivery
- Labour complications
- Delivery complications
- Birth trauma
- Medications
- Drug abuse
- Resuscitation

FOLLOWING BIRTH
- Ethnicity
- Gestation
- Geographical location
- Birth weight and weight gain
- Sepsis
- Family history
- Obstetric history
- Parental lifestyle choices
- Feeding
- Screening results
- Congenital abnormality
- Developmental abnormality
- Environmental factors
- Child protection issues

Socio-economic and demographic history

- **Ethnicity** – with health and nutritional status equal, outcomes do not vary by ethnicity (Villar *et al.,* 2014). Ethnic inequalities reduce fetal growth, birthweight, head and abdominal circumferences for Black and minority ethnicity (Louis *et al.,* 2015). Morbidity for age ≤1 year is highest for Black children (Green, 2012). Caucasians have slower lung maturation and higher respiratory disease than African-Americans or Filipinos (Haas *et al.,* 2011). Abnormalities vary; for example, dermal melanocytosis (Mongolian blue spot) – 75% in Asian, African, Mediterranean, Middle Eastern; 5% in Caucasian European.

- **National and international variations** – access to health support, education and genetics impact on morbidity and mortality (e.g. higher levels of spina bifida in Wales than the rest of the UK).
- **Age** – teenagers and advanced maternal age groups have increased adverse perinatal health and chromosomal abnormalities.
- **BMI/diet** – raised body mass index (BMI) is linked to neonatal macrosomia, birth trauma and hypoglycaemia. Low BMI impacts on attachment and feeding difficulties.
- **Substance abuse** – fetal alcohol syndrome or drug withdrawal and neonatal abstinence syndrome.

- **Smoker** – intrauterine growth retardation (IUGR), hypoxia, prematurity, hypertonia, irritability, increased risk of sudden infant death syndrome.
- **Economic constraints** – lower and middle income families have lower birth weight babies (Sletner *et al.*, 2013).
- **Consanguinity** – increases risk of congenital cardiac anomalies.
- **Domestic abuse and maternal child abuse** – increased risk of neonatal neglect, abuse or trauma in and following pregnancy.
- **Learning difficulties** – neonatal prematurity and low birth weight. Increased parental mental health issues, abuse and socio-economic deprivation and delayed development of parenting skills.

Family history

- **Sibling health** – reoccurrence likely (e.g. cardiac conditions increase 2–3% with one previous sibling, 50% with two siblings affected).
- **Relatives** (maternal or paternal) – risk increase related to any relative but particularly first degree relative with congenital or developed health concerns.
- **Child protection issues** – assess risk to neonate.

Screening and diagnostic results

- **Rhesus status, blood group and antibody results** – risk of haemolytic disease of the newborn (HDN), pathological jaundice.
- **HIV status** – preventative management reduces mother–child transmission to 1–2% but there is greater risk of other sexually transmitted infections, hepatitis, tuberculosis and neonatal toxaemia, anaemia and neutropenia.
- **Hepatitis** – risk of chronic hepatitis if not preventatively managed.
- **Rubella** – risk of congenital rubella syndrome.
- **Sickle cell** – risk of tissue hypoxia.
- **Thalassaemia** – risk of life-threatening anaemia.
- **Ultrasonography:**
  Dating scan – gestation, chromosomal abnormality (absent nasal bone);
  Nuchal translucency – chromosomal abnormality, 36% of congenital heart disease (Sotiriadis *et al.*, 2013);
  Ultrasound markers (echogenic bowel, ventriculomegaly, dilated renal pelves) – chromosomal abnormality and/or pathology;
  Growth scans – IUGR;
  Polyhydramnios – duodenal/oesophageal atresia;
  Oligohydramnios – premature rupture of membranes (PROM), growth restriction, infection, renal pathology;
  Fetal sex – sex-linked conditions.
- **Triple and quadruple tests** – chromosomal abnormalities.
- **Diagnostics** (amniocentesis, chorionic villi sampling, cordocentesis) – chromosomal abnormalities, isoimmunisation, trauma.

Medical and surgical history

- **Medical** – metabolic (diabetes, thyroidism), endocrine (pituitary or adrenal), renal, hypertension, cardiac, venereal, seizures.
- **Medication** – positive (folic acid), negative effects (thalidomide).

- **Psychological/psychiatric** – psychotropic medication withdrawal, fetal abnormalities (cardiac, neural tube, cleft palate, floppy baby syndrome), child protection.

Antenatal history

- **Delayed booking or poor attendance** – socio-economic risks greater.
- **Fundal height** – identification of reduced growth.
- **Presentation after 36 weeks' gestation** – breech presentation (even if vertex at birth) risk of developmental dysplasia of the hips (DDH).
- **Anti D** – HDN prevention; following antepartum haemorrhage.
- **Multiple pregnancy** – all risks increase.
- **Placental insufficiency** (haemorrhage, reduced movements, pre-eclampsia) – anoxia, meconium.
- **Infection** – risk of fetal infection (e.g. haemolytic streptococcus B, syphilis); or abnormality (e.g. rubella, cytomegalovirus, influenza).

Intrapartum and birth history

- **Maternal pyrexia and fetal tachycardia** – risk for neonatal infection.
- **Prelabour or prolonged rupture of membranes (PROM)** – the risk of serious neonatal infection is 1% (NICE, 2014).
- **Meconium liquor** – risk of meconium aspiration syndrome, respiratory compromise (NICE, 2014).
- **Presentation/position** – risk of DDH, trauma, adverse moulding.
- **Birth trauma** – risk of bruising, jaundice, nerve damage, bone fractures.
- **Precipitate delivery** – risk of tentorial tears, facial congestion.
- **Gestation** – prematurity, post maturity.
- **Fetal compromise** (blood gases, cardiac monitoring) – anoxia.
- **Instrumental/operative delivery** – risk of birth trauma, bruising, jaundice.
- **Medication** – antibiotic therapy (group B streptococcus), magnesium sulfate (hypermagnesaemia), reduced tone and inactivity, sodium – jaundice.

Early neonatal history

- **Apgar** – resuscitation, transition to extrauterine life.
- **Weight centile** – ≥90th (trauma, hypoglycaemia); ≤10th (IUGR).
- **Head circumference** – risk of microcephaly, hydrocephaly, abnormal moulding, cephalhaematoma, haemorrhage.
- **Signs of sepsis** – high, low or unstable temperature, respiratory problems, brady-/tachycardia, poor tone, poor feeding, unresponsive, seizures, jaundice, vomiting.
- **Screening results** (Kleihauer, Coombs, hearing, blood spot) – isoimmunisation, metabolic disorders, haemoglobinopathies.
- **Feeding** – hypoglycaemia, jaundice, dehydration, vomiting.
- **Bowel movements, urine stream** – physical abnormalities, renal disease, dehydration (urates), infection, feeding problems.

The relevant history and risk factors are summarised in Figure 25.1 from pre-pregnancy to the postnatal period.

26 Feeding

Box 26.1 Soft cues to demand feeding.

- Rapid eye movement (REM)
- Stirring from sleep
- Increased movements
- Fidgeting
- Rooting reflex seen
- Sucking reflex seen
- Sucking sounds heard
- Actual sucking of finger/hand

Box 26.2 Late cues (to be avoided).

Crying

⬇

Increasing distress

⬇

Newborn releasing cortisol (stress hormone)

Box 26.3 Signs of good latching.

- No pain on feeding
- Lying chest to chest
- Wide open mouth
- Lips curled out
- Areola fully in mouth (or more visible above than below)
- Head tilted back slightly
- Cheeks puffed out
- Sucking and swallowing
- Breasts emptying
- Weight gaining

Box 26.4 Decontamination of formula feeding equipment.

There are three main methods used for decontamination of formula feeding equipment:

1 Boiling
2 Chemical treatment
3 Steam (electrical or microwave)

Box 26.5 Essentials of formula feed preparation.

1 Clean/decontaminate all equipment
2 Wash hands and work surfaces
3 Make feeds one at a time as needed
4 Boil fresh tap water and leave to cool to 70°C (up to 30 mins)
5 Pour water in to bottle to correct level
6 Fill scoop provided with loose powder – do not compress; level off using knife
7 Add the correct number of scoops according to amount of water and age of baby
8 Secure teat without contaminating it
9 Add cap and shake to dissolve powder
10 Cool before feeding

Figure 26.1 Good latching. Source: Image courtesy of Tuomas_Lehtinen at FreeDigitalPhotos.net

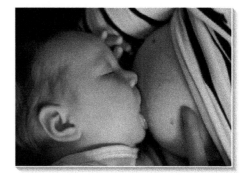

Physical Examination of the Newborn at a Glance, First Edition. Denise (Dee) Campbell and Lyn Dolby.
© 2018 John Wiley & Sons, Ltd. Published 2018 by John Wiley & Sons, Ltd.

The feeding decision will already have been made by the time of the physical examination. It is important that the examiner is not judgemental and respects individual choice with awareness that formula feeding may occur because of a contraindication to breastfeeding. This chapter concentrates on the assessment that feeding has been initiated/established and is progressing well, as well as recognition of the most common feeding problems.

Contraindications to breastfeeding

Sensitivity is required around situations in which breastfeeding may be the first choice but where breastfeeding (or milk production) is not possible, delayed or contraindicated. Additional support may be needed to express breast milk and establish a milk supply if breastfeeding is only delayed.

Maternal

- HIV infection;
- Antiretroviral medication;
- Human T-cell lymphotrophic virus types 1 and 2;
- Drug or substance abuse;
- Chemotherapy;
- Radiotherapy (treatment or diagnostic therapy);
- Active tuberculosis;
- Breast tissue damage (e.g. following trauma or breast augmentation);
- Bilateral mastectomy;
- Breast abscess;
- Active herpes simplex lesions on the breast;
- Active varicella zoster lesions on the breast;
- Coma.

Newborn

- Physical abnormality affecting the ability to feed (e.g. oesophageal atresia);
- Metabolic abnormality affecting tolerance to milk (e.g. galactosaemia, maple syrup urine disease, phenylketonuria);
- Acute illness or infection affecting the ability to feed;
- Prematurity.

Initiation and establishment of feeding

Positive signs – general

- Feeding commenced as soon after birth as possible.
- Demand feeding is practised associated with early feeding cues (Boxes 26.1 and 26.2).
- Newborn is waking naturally for feeds.
- Newborn is settling between feeds – cluster feeding is possible (a number of feeds in quick succession before a longer gap).
- No vomiting – dribbles and possets are possible.
- Normal micturition and stools – frequency, colour and consistency.
- Contented mother and newborn with evidence of bonding.
- Initial weight loss is no greater than 10% of birth weight and regaining from 4 days – back to or above birth weight by 14 days.
- No signs of newborn dehydration.

Breastfeeding specific

- Both breasts at each feed for unrestricted time period.
- 8–12 feeds per day.

- Progress from colostrum to milk by 24–72 hours.
- Filling of breasts between/before a feed (from 48–72 hours).
- Newborn latching well (Box 26.3 and Figure 26.1).
- Breasts emptying during feeds (4 days onwards).
- No supplementary feeding required.
- Nipples and breasts aproblematic.

Formula feeding specific

- 6–10 feeds per day and settling between feeds.
- Sucking and pausing are intermittent during feeds.
- Small feeds initially build to 150–200 mL/kg/day by 1 week old.
- Air flow back into bottle during paused feeding.
- Correct approaches to decontamination of equipment and making of feeds (Boxes 26.4 and 26.5).

Common problems

A full history should be taken around feeding including patterns, length, frequency, positioning of infant, air swallowing and winding. Examine for signs of infection, obstruction or ill health including frequency, colour, smell and amounts of urine and stool passed. If breastfeeding, examine the breasts for signs of infection or sore nipples. If formula feeding, assess decontamination of equipment, preparation and temperature of feed – by all individuals involved.

Excessive weight gain

This is weight gain above the expectation of a centile chart or where a significant jump is seen. Distinguish between correct demand feeding and incorrectly feeding whenever a newborn is fretful (as opposed to hungry). Over-concentrated formula, supplements, early weaning and over-feeding (pushing additional or longer feeds on an already satisfied newborn) can result in excessive weight gain.

Failure to thrive

This is inadequate weight gain after allowing for initial weight loss and variable weight gain patterns. A fall in weight gain is of greater concern than regular weight gain along a low centile. It may be caused by incorrect feeding (over-diluted feeds, poor latching), inadequate feeding (abuse or poor parenting), poor absorption (allergy or abnormality) or excessive elimination (diarrhoea or vomiting).

Vomiting

Small regurgitations or dribbles linked to feeding or winding are normal (possets). Errors in reconstitution of formula feeds, air swallowing, over-stimulation, over-feeding, infection, allergy, food intolerance, reflux, hernia or obstruction can lead to vomiting. It is important to assess the frequency, amount, colour and pattern of occurrence alongside the general health of the newborn.

Constipation

Passage of a hard dry stool. Infants may go 2–3 days without passing a stool and still not be constipated. Causes include dehydration, over-concentrated formula milk, incorrect feeding, stenosis (bowel or anus) or Hirschsprung's disease.

27 Excretion

Figure 27.1 Meconium.
Source: Jeremy Kemp - English Wikipedia, Copyrighted free use, https://commons.wikimedia.org/w/index.php?curid=1658551.

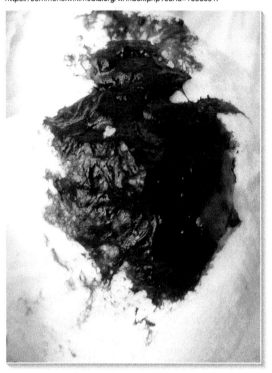

Figure 27.2 Changing stool.
Source: Belgaman at Dutch Wikipedia https://upload.wikimedia.org/wikipedia/commons/b/bc/Diaper_Contents_after_user.jpg. Licensed under CC-BY-SA-3.0.

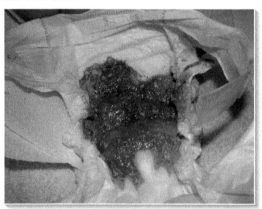

Box 27.1 Symptoms of urinary tract infection – some or all may be present.

- Hot to touch/pyrexia
- Not eating as well as normal
- Vomiting
- Irritability/pain on handling
- Cloudy, blood-stained, darker urine
- More sleepy than normal
- Diarrhoea (difficult to determine if breastfed – note changes from normal)
- More offensive stool

Figure 27.3 Breastfed stool.
Source: By Tradimus (Own work) [CC0], via Wikimedia Commons. https://commons.wikimedia.org/wiki/File%3ANeonatal_stool.jpg9.

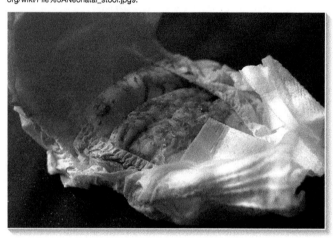

Figure 27.4 Artificial fed stool – semi-formed.

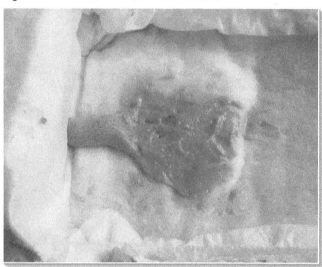

Figure 27.5 Hydronephrosis (level 1 left; level 4 right).

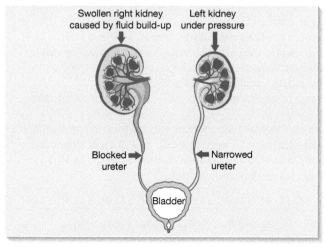

Swollen right kidney caused by fluid build-up

Left kidney under pressure

Blocked ureter

Narrowed ureter

Bladder

Physical Examination of the Newborn at a Glance, First Edition. Denise (Dee) Campbell and Lyn Dolby.
© 2018 John Wiley & Sons, Ltd. Published 2018 by John Wiley & Sons, Ltd.

This chapter details normal excretion and includes information about the more common problems that may occur, their symptoms and their causes. The focus is on excretion from the bladder and bowel (abnormal excretion from the mouth, nose and lungs is included in their specific chapters). The relevant history and risk factors should be considered before examination: family history, anomaly screening, oligohydramnios and meconium liquor. The examination benefits from knowledge of normal genitalia, patency of the external anal meatus, kidney palpation and details of the feeding pattern. It is essential that the number and nature of bladder and bowel movements is ascertained, as well as any vomiting or abdominal distension preceding the examination.

Bowel

In utero, from 16 weeks' gestation, meconium has formed in the colon. A mixture of epithelial, amniotic and blood cells within the digestive tract, along with mucus, bile, amniotic fluid and fatty acids, have been acted upon by digestive enzymes, resulting in this greeny-black substance (Figure 27.1). The presence of meconium helps to keep the colon patent along its length as the fetus grows. Unlike the bladder, the bowel is not typically active in utero. Meconium may be passed by the post mature fetus or during episodes of fetal compromise. Reduced oxygen levels cause muscle relaxation, including the anal sphincter and meconium escapes into the liquor.

The consistency of any meconium in the liquor changes over time, becoming more diluted – this is affected by the amount and time of meconium passed. Degrees and consistency of meconium are classified as significant (dark green–black, thick or tenacious, or containing lumps) or insignificant and management in utero, at birth and postnatally is determined accordingly (NICE, 2014).

Typically, meconium is first passed in the 24 hours following birth and clears from the system in approximately 48 hours. By day 2–3 a green–brown, changing stool becomes evident (Figure 27.2). This is when the lighter coloured stool of the feeding baby appears seedy and stained from the traces of meconium. After this the stool is affected by the type of feeding:

- **Breastfeeding** (Figure 27.3) – loose, bright yellow–green, inoffensive and often with a mustard seed appearance. Huge range in frequency is normal from 1 stool every 3 days to 10 per day.
- **Artificial feeding** (Figure 27.4) – pale, semi-formed, with a sour smell. Frequency is 4–6 per day, with increased risk of firm or constipated stool.

Abnormalities

- **Constipation** – difficulties passing firm stool. Infrequent passage of stool is rarely constipation unless accompanied by severe straining, anal twitching and signs of discomfort. Increase fluids and breastfeed more frequently; check artificial feed mix.
- **Delayed passage of stool** – consider meconium plug, meconium ileus, Hirschsprung's disease, cystic fibrosis and imperforate anus.
- **Diarrhoea** – increased frequency and runniness of stool. May be a result of infection, maternal diet, fore–hind milk imbalance, food allergy.

- **Haematochezia** – fresh blood in stool. May be linked to food allergies from mother (lactose intolerance), infection or fissures caused by constipation.
- **Melaena** – partially digested blood from upper digestive tract in stool; stool appears black (after meconium stage).
- **Mucus** – can be normal in a breastfeeding baby. If it persists, ensure fore and hind milk are taken in balance and consider food allergy to something the mother is eating.
- **Pus** – white cells in a microbiology tested stool; result of inflammation or infection.
- **White stool** – may be caused by a medication taken. Also, consider anaemia, lack of bile, cyst or tumour, lactose intolerance or galactosaemia.

Kidneys and bladder

Bladder filling and emptying begins in utero for the normal healthy newborn but the placenta remains the organ of excretion. The kidneys remain immature at birth, rapidly maturing over the first week. Poor glomerular filtration initially causes difficulties in concentrating the urine (with reabsorption of sodium and imbalanced fluid loss) and may result in urine having a cloudy appearance at birth. Micturition for the newborn is a basic reflex controlled by the spinal cord in response to stretching of the trigone within the bladder. The trigone is a sensitive triangle in the wall of the bladder between the two ureters and urethra. At birth, as little as 35–75 mL urine will be passed each day (Sinha *et al.*, 2012), rising to approximately 200 mL/day by 10 days.

The first urine passed is normally within 24 hours and would typically be pale, straw-coloured and inoffensive. A reddish-brown, powdery discharge (urates) sometimes occurs as a result of mild dehydration, slight acidosis (uric acid) or fluid imbalance. This is insignificant unless it continues beyond the first few days. Occasionally, there may even be no urine passed in the first 48 hours but if the infant is alert, feeding well and there is no vomiting nor abdominal swelling, this is unlikely to be a problem. It may be just that urine has been missed within the stool of a dirty nappy but, a square of kitchen roll or tissue placed in the nappy will help monitor urine output.

Abnormalities

- **Hydronephrosis** (Figure 27.5) – fluid filling the kidney. This is caused by blockage or restricted flow of urine away from the kidney – most commonly a narrowed ureter. May resolve spontaneously after birth but severe cases require surgery.
- **Haematuria** – blood in urine. Visible blood should not be present. Investigation is needed for signs of renal failure, infection (Box 27.1), tumour, trauma or coagulation disorders.
- **Oliguria** – failure to make and/or pass urine. Caused by developmental complication, obstruction, neurological damage, renal agenesis or cardiopulmonary disease.
- **Urine dribbling/leakage** – because of posterior urethral valves (male infants only). Partial blockage of the urethra leads to an enlarged bladder under pressure and slowly dribbling urine. Untreated, back flow damage can cause renal failure.

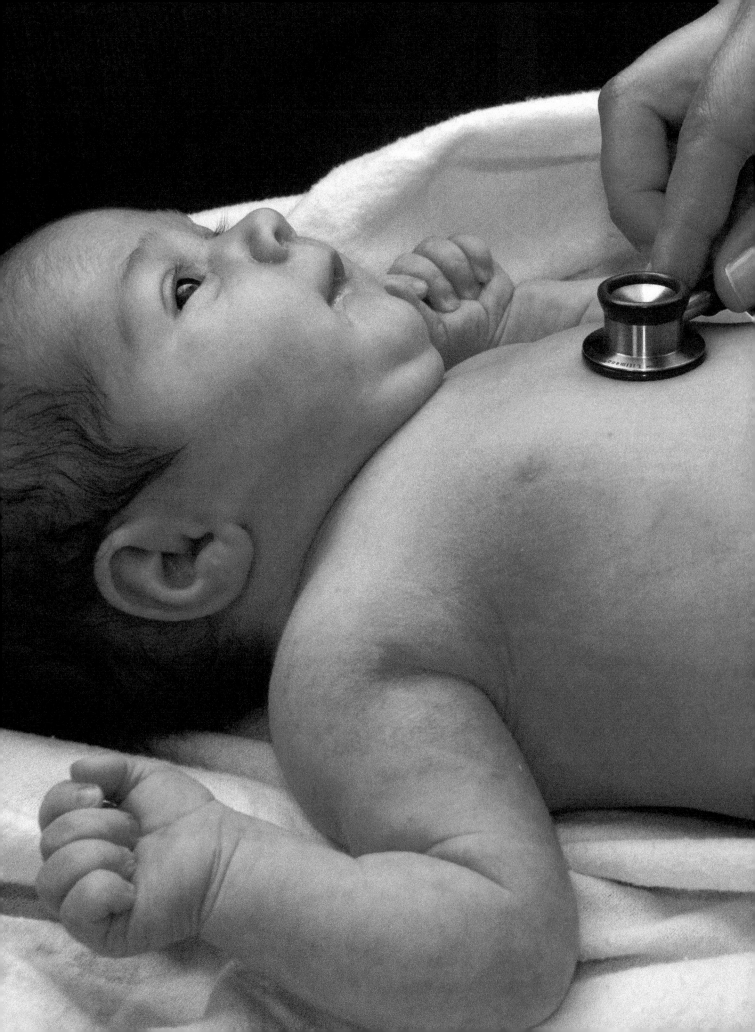

Top to toe physical examination

Part 5

Chapters

28 Newborn and infant physical examination – overview

Table 28.1 Key aspects of the newborn and infant physical examination.

Aspect	Observe and assess the following elements	
Colour	Pink or well perfused	Jaundiced? Transcutaneous reading obtained or SBR taken? Results?
Head	Skull and fontanelles Facial features and ears/signs of dysmorphia Hearing screening performed?	Head circumference Appropriate use of tape measure (cm towards brow) to aid consistency of measurement
Neck/clavicles	Tumours, webbing, fractures	
Palate	Digital and visual inspection:	Teeth, tongue and/or lip tie
Posture/behaviour	Flexion, tone, response to touch and handling Alertness and general demeanour	
Cardiac	Use an infant-sized stethoscope and auscultate with both diaphragm and bell Apex rate: cap. refill and thrills	Brachial and femoral pulses Pedal pulses (if required) Cord bloods taken? – results?
Respiratory	Rate noted, clear air entry?	Recession, grunting, nasal flaring
Chest	Shape Nipples	Neonatal gynaecomastia
Abdomen	Masses, tone	Kidneys palpated
Umbilicus	Clamp secure, on	Inflammation/discharge Hernia
Upper limbs	No. of digits counted L and R Palm creases	Bone integrity Movement, interdigital webbing
Lower limbs	Bone integrity No. of digits: L and R Plantar creases	Movement Talipes Interdigital webbing
Genitalia	*Male* Epstein's pearls, epispadias Smooth urine flow Penis length/chordee Hydrocele, testes ↓↓	*Female* Appearance Pseudomenstruation Mucous Tags
Hips	Allis sign – leg length Thigh and buttock creases	Ortolani and Barlow's manoeuvres: L and R = 'stable'? Single hip anomaly – note if 'unstable' or 'dislocated', etc.
Spine	Integrity (link with how baby moves arms and legs)	Sacral dimple/hair tufts Naevus/abnormal skin patches
Eyes	Appearance Discharge: sticky or purulent Alert, fixation	Red reflex normal: L and R noted as normal Use of ophthalmoscope Subconjunctival haemorrhage or trauma from delivery
Skin	Condition Rashes	Birth marks Trauma
Anus	Appearance, position Patency	Meconium passed and date Changing stool or unusual consistency (e.g. pale, green)
Urine	Urine passed and date noted (link with abdominal findings)	Urates passed
Reflexes	Suckling, gag and blink Moro (noted if bilateral and equal) Incurving (Galant reflex)	Stepping/placing Grasp Babinski/plantar flexion
Vaccination	Anti-D; BCG required or given?	
Feeding	Method, frequency and progress	If artificial formula – which one? Quantity?
Health promotion information	Immunisations Parental health activities – car seats, pram systems, smoking, safer sleeping and 'tummy time' Signs of ill health and where to seek advice Next screening examination with the GP	

Physical Examination of the Newborn at a Glance, First Edition. Denise (Dee) Campbell and Lyn Dolby.
© 2018 John Wiley & Sons, Ltd. Published 2018 by John Wiley & Sons, Ltd.

At times, an abnormality that was not detected during pregnancy or soon after birth presents during the neonatal period even in an apparently healthy baby. Occasionally, one of the parents voices a concern about a particular issue, or during the examination the practitioner finds an anomaly. At these moments, the level of professional sensitivity, knowledge and understanding employed will make a significant difference to the parents as the initial impact of the issue of concern sinks in. However, it is paramount that if anomalies are found these concerns must be expressed to the parents followed by an explanation regarding the action that will be taken. It should never be the case that a particular anomaly, or specific signs and symptoms, are noted and the baby referred to the paediatric team without discussing the findings with the parents – this would be wholly unacceptable practice.

The assessment of neonatal health and well-being commences with the initial examination at birth and continues with the daily examination of the baby. The National Screening Programme (Public Health England, 2016a) examination of the newborn offers screening for all babies within 72 hours of birth. The examination is offered again at the 6–8 week examination with the GP. If there is any cause for concern between these two examinations, parents should have been informed during the earlier examination who they should contact for an urgent concern as opposed to a more minor issue.

Under normal circumstances, this examination should be offered within 72 hours of birth. If the baby becomes ill and conducting the examination is not feasible, it must be noted clearly and the next member of staff that cares for the baby must be informed that the examination has not yet been performed.

There are certain criteria concerning who can complete the examination, depending on the condition, age or already identified concerns. For example, midwives who have received further training (either post registration or as part of the initial pre-registration midwifery programme of study) to enable them to conduct the examination of the newborn can do so only for babies who are ≥37 weeks' gestation or who have reached a particular centile by birth. The local protocols and guidelines for the practice area must be taken into account and it is the practitioner's responsibility to be fully conversant with these.

Pre-examination

The practitioner should investigate the notes for predisposing factors, maternal blood results and identification of conditions that have already been noted and the management specified. At times, this information will mean that the baby must be examined by a member of the paediatric team and the parents need to be made aware of this.

As with all examinations, the parent(s) should always be informed about what the examination process entails, their understanding of this assessed and their ability to understand the language used by the practitioner also needs to be determined. This is not only so that the parent(s) can make an informed decision in relation to consent, but they also need to understand the examination findings and the information that is shared with them throughout the examination. Sometimes it is necessary to obtain the services of an interpreter and most Trusts have a service to support this.

The examination should be performed where it can be easily witnessed by the parent(s) and the lighting is good, preferably in natural daylight (easier to detect cyanosis, some birthmarks and level of jaundice). Hands should be washed and dried prior to the examination and everything required should be close at hand (e.g.

nappy and baby clothes). The examination should be performed quickly and comprehensively, only uncovering the part of the baby being examined and re-covering the baby as soon as is practicable in order that he/she does not become unduly cold and fretful. The examiner should be professional and gentle in his/her actions; no parent likes to see their baby's arms and legs used as 'handles'. The stethoscope or ophthalmoscope should not be placed in the cot with the baby or the nappy removed and placed near the baby's head as both are aspects of poor infection control.

It is necessary to remember that parents observe the examiner's actions, facial expressions and the words used and how they are spoken. Therefore, if the baby is fidgety and it is taking a while to perform auscultation of the heart, reassure the parents. Likewise, if the examiner finds an anomaly, it should be discussed with the parents at the time and, if no immediate action is necessary, return to the issue again at the end of the examination, summarising what will happen next.

Examination of the newborn – process

The examination of the newborn should include the aspects and elements identified in Table 28.1, and should follow a systematic process in order not to miss any part of the examination. Always commence the examination by asking the parent(s) for their impression of their baby's health and if they have any concerns as these may include issues that have arisen during the antenatal period. Parents should also be asked if they have any family history of heart, kidney or hip conditions from birth, as occasionally something that has become 'normal' for the parent(s) is not highlighted at booking.

It is always best to commence the examination with auscultation of the heart (if the baby is calm) and then continue with a top to toe examination. This allows the hands to be in gentle contact with the baby most of the time, allowing the baby to gradually wake and preventing over-stimulation. Certain aspects of the examination such as auscultation of the heart, eye examination and hip assessment can prove impossible with a crying baby. Sometimes the examination should be temporarily abandoned if the baby is too distressed until the reason for the distress is resolved (e.g. pain, needs feeding).

Examining the eyes sometimes proves difficult as at this stage of life the baby, unless fully alert, is more likely to keep his/her eyes closed or only partly open. Use of the doll's eye reflex, placing the baby over the mother's shoulder or on her knee or even walking into a darker area of the room and closing the curtains can help. A baby who is gently spoken to will tend to be calmer and more alert as he/she concentrates on the source of vocalisation.

The hip assessment usually occurs just before the baby is gently picked up and turned over in order to view the back and elicit the walking/pacing reflexes. On turning the baby over, perform the reflexes first as some babies become accustomed to lying over the hand when their back is examined and are then reluctant to demonstrate the reflexes.

Post examination

Feeding and health education can be discussed, including any issues such as unilateral undescended testes which will be reassessed during the 6–8 week examination. The parent(s) should be fully informed of the findings of the examination and if issues of concern have arisen, what will happen next or if action needs to be taken urgently. All findings should be documented in full within the neonatal record, the Trust digital system, the SMART system and the Personal Child Health Record.

29 # Neurological assessment

Table 29.1 Normal stages of sleep state.

Sleep state	Sleep	Baby's movements/activity
State 1	Deep sleep	Regular breathing, eyes closed with no eye movement visible, no spontaneous activity but may make regular jerky movements. External stimuli produces slightly delayed startle motion which is rapidly suppressed
State 2	Light sleep (active sleep)	Eyes are closed, but rapid eye movements are visible with the eyes opening for a brief moment. Baby makes random movements and often responds to internal and external stimuli which often provoke a change in sleep state. Respiration can be irregular and suckling movements occur intermittently
State 3	Drowsy (semi-dozing)	Eyes may be open, but any response to external stimuli is delayed. However, sleep state may change after stimuli. Slight startles may occur, but movement is smooth
State 4	Quiet awake	Baby is alert, focused and attentive. Other stimulus may distract the focus of attention but the response is delayed. Motor activity is minimal. Learning activity is high
State 5	Fussing	Eyes are open with considerable bodily activity. Reacts to external stimuli with increased activity. Fussy vocalisation may be heard, may quieten to sound of mother's voice or cuddling
State 6	Crying	Intense crying with lots of activity. May take time to quieten with cuddling or consoling activities

Box 29.1 Key neurological alarm signals.

- Persistent irritability
- Difficulty in feeding
- Persistent deviation of head or eyes
- Asymmetry in posture and movements that is persistent
- Opisthotonus
- Floppiness
- Abnormal cry
- Apathy or conversely hyperexcitability and jitteriness
- Convulsions
- Setting-sun sign
- Respiratory difficulties, apnoea, changes of loss of variability in heart rate

Box 29.2 Congenital malformations of the brain.

- Anencephaly
- Cranial encephalocele and meningocele
- Spina bifida (occulta)
- Meningocele
- Myelomeningocele
- Hydrocephalus and hydranencephaly
- Dandy–Walker syndrome
- Agenesis of corpus callosum
- Megalencephaly
- Microcephaly

Physical Examination of the Newborn at a Glance, First Edition. Denise (Dee) Campbell and Lyn Dolby.
© 2018 John Wiley & Sons, Ltd. Published 2018 by John Wiley & Sons, Ltd.

Good observational skills are important when assessing the normal neurological responses in a baby. It is important to take time to note how the baby responds to handling and other stimuli such as sound and light.

Sleep patterns

Although the preterm baby may spend much of his/her time asleep, the cycles between activity and rest, regular and irregular breathing and whether eye movements are visible is not so pronounced as in a term baby. This reflects the latter's maturity, not just physically but also mentally.

The normal term baby will usually move between behavioural states, spending most of his/her time in quiet and active sleep. Approximately 50 minutes per hour will consist of sleep time, of which 50% will be spent in quiet sleep. Brazelton and Nugent (2011) define the normal sleep pattern as passing through a number of stages or 'states' unless this pattern is interrupted, for example by the baby being picked up (Table 29.1).

Body position and activity

The normal body posture for a baby, whether prone or supine, is well flexed with the head usually lying in the midline and limbs often held in a roughly symmetrical position. Babies with intact neurology often alternately move their arms and legs. As both palmar and plantar grasp are present in the fetus from 26 weeks' gestation (grasp reflex persists until approximately 4 months of age) and therefore by term the hands are usually tightly closed and often held near the chin or upper part of the body.

Many babies may appear to 'jitter' or startle in their sleep (Table 29.1), but one can easily test if this is normal movement (known as a myoclonic jerk) as opposed to a seizure by holding the limb in question – if it is a normal movement the jitter will stop. With a seizure this will not happen and it may be accompanied by ocular deviation or autonomic changes, such as mottling, or changes in colour or respiratory rate.

When the baby's limbs are moved, there should be obvious muscle resistance and tone. If the baby is pulled to sitting position, the head may initially lag slightly but the baby should be able to demonstrate movement towards the upright position. The baby may not be able to hold his/her own head up for long, but the ability to do so has been demonstrated.

When lying in ventral suspension over the examiner's hand, the baby should be capable of holding head and legs in alignment with the back. This may only be for a short time as a sleepy baby may not demonstrate this ability. The baby should also be capable of flexing his/her limbs against gravity.

Demonstrating the neurological reflexes that are present in the newborn baby are important in enabling the parents to see what their baby is capable of and to learn why. However, these reflexes are also important in assessing the integrity of the neurological system (for further information, see Chapter 30).

Crying

Crying is a baby's method of communicating with the world as he/she tries to convey discomfort, hunger or pain. A normal healthy term baby will have a lusty cry which eventually terminates when appropriate method of solace is given, such as being cuddled close to the chest or over the parent's shoulder. However, it is abnormal for a baby to have a persistent high-pitched or weak cry and this may demonstrate that there is a neurological impact caused, for example, by drug withdrawal or hypoxic–ischaemic encephalopathy.

Feeding and suckling

Some neurologically sound babies may not want to feed because of a headache caused by trauma experienced during birth. However, the rooting reflex is present by 28 weeks' gestation and suckling begins during week 11, with the ability to coordinate suckling and swallowing at approximately 28 weeks' gestation. Strength and coordination of breathing occurs around 32–34 weeks' gestation. Therefore, if the baby does not appear capable of normal feeding responses, the integrity of the cranial nerves should be tested. The practitioner can try to elicit the rooting reflex by gently stroking the upper lip or corner of the mouth. The fifth cranial nerve is involved here as this conducts sensation; nerves 5, 7 and 12 relate to the motor pathways, and swallowing involves nerves 9 and 10. If suckling is absent, the practitioner can test the gag reflex by gently stroking the soft palate with a cotton bud, which should elicit the appropriate response.

Eyes

A pupillary reflex (pupil reacts to light) is often apparent in the fetus after 30 weeks, but always by 35 weeks' gestation. Even a baby of 26 weeks' gestation will respond to light by blinking and can briefly track objects by 34 weeks. Therefore, how the eyes of a term baby react to light, how they move and fixate can provide important neurological markers.

The pupils of the eyes will usually lie mid position and will generally move together in the same direction. Horizontal divergence is normal until about 6 weeks of age, when the activity of looking and focusing on objects should have provided enough stimuli to strengthen the muscles of the eye and nerve pathways. However, abnormal reactions include constant deviation and persistent strabismus or nystagmus. It is important to note here that vertical deviation is always abnormal, often the result of germinal matrix haemorrhage or intraventricular haemorrhage. Although both of these types of haemorrhage are more likely to occur in preterm babies, it is not unknown for them to occur in the term neonate.

Neurological alarm signals

Box 29.1 presents a list of the most common signs that all is not well in relation to neurological function. The main causes of neurological compromise requiring referral and/or investigation include the following.

- **Seizures** – most start 12–48 hours after birth, with 50% caused by hypoxic–ischaemic encephalopathy, or to a lesser extent focal cerebral infarction or viral or bacterial infection.
- **Meningitis** – current incidence is 0.25–0.5 per 1000 births.
- **Drug withdrawal** – symptoms can occur up to 3 weeks after birth, effects can persist for several months; withdrawal from methadone is worse than from heroin.
- **Intracranial haemorrhage** – seizures are usually noted and sometimes pyrexia.
- **Hypoxic–ischaemic brain injury** – usually caused by a hypoxic episode during the intrapartum period.
- **Acidosis** – from respiratory failure or metabolic in origin.
- **Hypoglycaemia** – more likely in babies who are small for their gestational age and effect is heightened with hypoxia.
- **Hypocalcaemia and hyponatraemia**.
- **Congenital malformations of the brain** (Box 29.2).
- **Hereditary and degenerative central nervous system disease**.
- **Inborn errors of metabolism** – phenylketonuria (PKU) and galactosaemia.
- **Congenital brain tumours** – most common is astrocytoma.
- **Cerebrovascular malformations** – such as Sturge–Weber syndrome.

30 Reflexes

Table 30.1 Reflexes usually assessed during the examination of the newborn.

Present by/established by	Primitive reflex	Disappears by approximately
28/32 weeks	Palmar flexion (grasp)	2–4 months
28/34 weeks	Rooting	3–4 months
28/40 weeks	Suck	4–6 months
32 weeks	Plantar flexion	8–12 months
32 weeks	Moro/startle	2–4 months
34 weeks	Babinski	9–12 months
35–37 weeks	Step	3 months but returns at approximately 9 months
35–37 weeks	Placing	Permanent
Birth	Blinking	Permanent
35/40	Gag	Permanent
Birth	Incurving or Galant	3–6 months
Birth	Swallow	Permanent
Birth	Ventral suspension	–

Figure 30.1 Babinski's reflex.

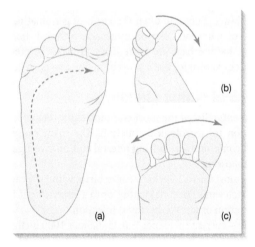

(a)   (b)   (c)

Figure 30.2 Plantar flexion.

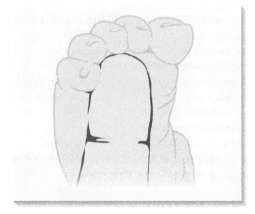

Figure 30.3 Eliciting the Moro reflex.
Source: Sinha *et al*. (2012). Reproduced with permission of John Wiley & Sons.

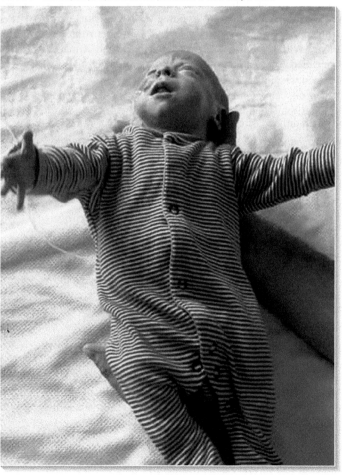

Physical Examination of the Newborn at a Glance, First Edition. Denise (Dee) Campbell and Lyn Dolby.
© 2018 John Wiley & Sons, Ltd. Published 2018 by John Wiley & Sons, Ltd.

Neonatal reflexes

More than 70 developmental reflexes have been identified (Illingworth, 1987), with some originating as simple spinal cord responses whereas others are far more complicated requiring interaction between the brain and other developing nerve centres. However, many of the primary reflexes (Table 30.1) that can be assessed at birth were initiated during intrauterine life and are often referred to as primitive, locomotor and postural reflexes.

Primitive reflexes are involuntary (not learned) and are essential for neonatal survival: rooting; suckling; swallowing; urinating; grasp; and Moro reflex. *Locomotor* reflexes link to the development of later voluntary movement; for example, the step reflex will develop later into 'walking'. Many of the *postural* reflexes develop after approximately 3 months of age and are therefore termed secondary reflexes, but the tonic neck reflex is observable at birth.

Assessment

During the the examination of the newborn, the following reflexes tend to be observed or elicited as the top to toe examination progresses. However, particular reflexes (e.g. Moro and rooting reflexes) may occur spontaneously and a mental note that they have been observed should be made at the time.

It is easier to elicit or observe responses if the baby is calm and not agitated. Parents are usually very interested in learning what their baby is capable of and the process of their child's development.

Rooting, suck, gag and swallow

If the cheek or corner of the mouth is stroked or touched, the baby will start to open his/her mouth and turn towards the stimulus. Touching or stroking of the lips will encourage the baby to open his/her mouth wider, allowing a finger or nipple to enter and further encourage *suckling*, allowing assessment of strength and coordination. Swallowing movements can be seen and the gag reflex may be elicited when exploring for integrity of the soft palate.

Head lag

Head lag is not usually routinely performed on a term baby. The baby's arms or hands are held securely whilst he/she is raised to a sitting position. The head will momentarily support itself in the midline and will then lag to one side or fall backward. Eventually, full head control will be achieved as the neck muscles strengthen.

Ventral suspension and incurving (Galant)

A demonstration of ventral suspension can be elicited when the term baby is placed tummy downwards over the hand and his/her arms and legs flex in conjunction with the head lifting and rotating. Incurving or the Galant reflex will be observed if a finger is gently drawn down one side of the body causing the baby's pelvis to curve to the side being tested. Both of these reflexes assist in the development of crawling movements.

Blinking

Blinking, as in adults, serves to protect the eye from trauma by distributing moisture around the eye and softening the impact of direct contact with objects. Any neurological impact that prevents the eye from closing such as facial nerve palsy will require administration of lubrication (artificial tears) to prevent corneal damage.

Tonic neck reflex ('fencing position')

When the infant is in a supine, neutral position, turn his/her head to one side. The arm on the side the head is turned to will extend (often with the hand opening), whilst flexion occurs in the opposite arm and leg. The reflex disappears at approximately 2–4 months of age. An inability or exaggerated response can indicate an abnormality.

Palmar flexion (grasp)

Stroking the palm of the baby's hand with a finger should stimulate palmar flexion which becomes stronger when an attempt is made to withdraw the finger. The strength of the palmar grasp can be assessed by the practitioner pulling their finger towards themselves and observing that the baby's body can lift off the bed.

Babinski's reflex and plantar flexion

Babinski's reflex will usually occur as a natural progression after plantar flexion has been elicited. The former response is encouraged by drawing the examiner's finger towards the little toe and across the ball of the foot (Figure 30.1a). The toes will extend and flex toward the dorsum of the foot (Figure 30.1b) whilst splaying apart (Figure 30.1c). If the reflex is consistently absent, it may point to an underlying neurological abnormality. The plantar reflex is easily elicited by applying finger pressure to the ball of the foot just under the toe line causing a flexion of the toes towards the plantar surface (Figure 30.2). Plantar flexion assists with crawling but disappears to allow the development of stable walking which cannot easily occur if the toes are flexed.

Moro or startle

The baby should be calm and supported in a supine, neutral position with his/her hands close to his/her body (Figure 30.3). The examiner tilts the baby's head forward towards its chest and then suddenly allows the head to drop backward a couple of centimetres. Initially, the baby's response will be to quickly extend and abduct his/her arms and the hands will open with the fingers splaying apart. This action will be followed by a slight adduction with accompanying flexion and closing of the hands. Complete absence of this reflex is abnormal and asymmetric movements may suggest brachial plexus palsy or a bone injury. However, it is possible for the Moro reflex to be elicited in the event of clavicular fracture where the bone ends are in good apposition to one another causing little discomfort to the baby.

Stepping and placing

Observing one or other of these reflexes is usually regarded as a positive response. Stepping is best elicited immediately after turning the baby from the supine position to the 'standing' position with the baby's body slightly leaning forward. Contact between the baby's feet and a flat surface should encourage alternate stepping movements. Placing is best elicited by the examiner holding the baby round the top of his/her trunk in an upright, suspended position. The baby is slowly raised until the dorsum of the foot touches a protruding edge (often the edge of a cot). In response to this stimulus the baby will purposefully flex his/her hip and knee and lift (or place) the foot on top of the protruding surface.

Abnormal findings

Generally, reflexes that are overly exaggerated or where there is an inability to elicit the required response can indicate the presence of an abnormality. However, one should first check that other factors are not affecting the baby. For example, the baby may be agitated and wanting to feed, may be affected by maternal drugs (e.g. pethidine) or the aftermath of a traumatic birth. Repeating the neurological assessment when the baby is calm and comfortable would be advantageous.

In the event of any abnormal findings, referral to the neonatologist should be expedited and a comprehensive record of the details should be completed within the neonatal record. Parents will need time with the neonatologist in order to discuss the findings and any future investigations that may be required.

31 Common skin conditions

Figure 31.1 (a) Erythema toxicum neonatorum. (b) Harlequin colour change. (c) Cutis marmorata.
Source: Irvine *et al.* (2011). Reproduced with permission of John Wiley & Sons.

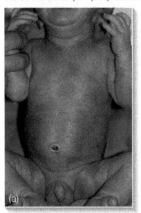

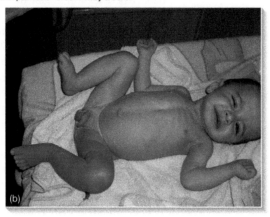

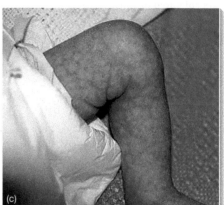

(a)   (b)   (c)

Table 31.1 Common terms used to describe skin conditions.

Erythema	Patches of skin with superficial reddening
Macule	Flat, dark area on the skin
Naevus	A raised birthmark
Papule	Pimple or spot
Pustule	Papule filled with pus
Vesicle	Fluid-filled bubble

Table 31.2 Rash type conditions that commonly occur during the first 2 weeks of life.

Condition	Appearance		Management/treatment
Erythema toxicum neonatorum	Small, firm, white–yellow pustules with an erythematous base, appearing between 1 and 2 days post birth	(Figure 31.1a)	No treatment required and the condition will usually self-resolve within a week of life
Milia	Occurs in 50% of newborn babies, presenting as small (1–2 mm in size), white pearly keratin vesicles of 1–2 mm in size on the face or scalp		No treatment required, usually resolves spontaneously after a few weeks
Sebaceous gland hyperplasia	Multiple white and yellow papules, commonly on the cheeks, upper lips and forehead, where sebaceous gland cells are most numerous. Develops as a response to the influence of maternal hormonal influences on the pilosebaceous follicles		No treatment required, usually resolves spontaneously within a few months
Nappy rash	Caused by prolonged exposure to stools and urine, rubbing of nappies, use of soaps or detergents. May occur as a consequence of illness or diarrhoea. The skin in the nappy area may become inflamed and/or develop spots, pustules or blisters		Frequent nappy changes, cleansing from front to back with plain water or newborn baby wipes. Only apply barrier cream sparingly. Leaving the area uncovered, but keeping the baby warm may also help
Neonatal seborrhoeic dermatitis	'Cradle cap'. Possibly caused by overactive sebaceous glands stimulated by maternal hormones. Presents as inflammation and greasy scales usually form on the scalp, and a non-irritating rash may sometimes extend to the face, ears, neck, flexures and nappy area. Milder cases may resolve within a few weeks without treatment. If necessary, frequent shampoos and gently removing the softened scales may help, or applying an emollient overnight before washing the scalp. If it does not demonstrate signs of resolving – refer the baby		An antifungal shampoo and mild topical corticosteroid can be prescribed

Physical Examination of the Newborn at a Glance, First Edition. Denise (Dee) Campbell and Lyn Dolby.
© 2018 John Wiley & Sons, Ltd. Published 2018 by John Wiley & Sons, Ltd.

The newborn skin

The functions of human skin are multifactorial in that it provides a mechanical barrier against microorganisms and toxins if intact. The thickness of the stratum corneum (the outerlayer of the skin) has an important part in thermoregulation and reducing fluid loss. Communication and learning are enhanced as a result of the sensory input derived from the nerve endings within the dermis.

However, the skin of a newborn baby is immature, alkaline and not yet colonised by the normal fauna and flora that assists in the protection against harmful bacteria. During the third trimester of pregnancy, amniotic fluid and vernix (discarded cells from the stratum corneum) raise the acidity of the stratum corneum. The level of vernix on the baby's skin has usually reduced by birth, but it acts as a natural cleanser and moisturiser and is an anti-infective and antioxidant, so it is important to not to try to remove the vernix from the baby unless it sits in large clumps which will attract dust and dirt. By approximately 5 days of age, the skin of the term infant has become more acidic and the uppermost layer has become drier and less vulnerable, both of which help to protect the neonate from infection (Jackson, 2008).

The thickness of the stratum corneum varies depending on the age of the baby, but in a term infant it is only 30% of the depth of that of an adult. This allows for greater permeability which may not only cause excessive dryness through water loss, but can also allow for easier absorption of chemicals from any cream or lotion that is applied (Crozier and Macdonald, 2010). At term, the dermis is only 60% of the depth of that in an adult. Therefore, traumatic delivery or scratches from an amniohook or scalp electrode can cause a breech in the skin barrier through which infection can enter.

Skin care and use of skin preparations

The aim of skin care is to avoid injury and prevent excessive dryness which can cause cracking and fissures, particularly around the wrists, which may lead to infection. Parents should understand the risk associated with using creams and lotions on their baby's skin. Parents should be advised to use plain water for bathing. If cleansing is required, only a mild, non-perfumed soap should be used (NICE, 2015). The prolonged effects of using oils to lubricate neonatal skin have not yet been comprehensively researched and are therefore not advised (Cooke et al., 2015).

Skin problems in neonates are quite common, but most of the time they are benign and will resolve relatively quickly. However, there are some skin conditions and birthmarks that can pose a significant risk to health. The role of practitioners is to inspect the neonatal skin regularly and be able to identify the more common neonatal skin lesions and those that warrant medical referral. Parents will often need comprehensive information and discussion even with those skin conditions that are frequently observed in neonates.

Common skin conditions – birth to 14 days

The conditions and birthmarks that appear during the first 2 weeks of life include conditions such as those of a physiological origin, non-infective (often transient), vascular and/or developmental, inheritable and inflammatory conditions. The chapters on neonatal skin focus on the more common conditions that may present themselves during the first 2 weeks. Some of the terms commonly used to describe the appearance of a skin condition can be seen in Table 31.1.

Cysts, papules and vesicles

Practitioners need to appreciate the differing appearance of various skin conditions and their management (Table 31.2).

Erythema toxicum neonatorum is thought to occur as a defensive mechanism as each papule contains eosinophils. The papules appear primarily on the face and trunk, each one visible for a few hours and then another appears in a different location. The condition is usually only visible during the time it takes the skin to become more acidic and develop the natural fauna and flora of extrauterine life, but occasionally will last up to 2 weeks.

Milia and **sebaceous gland hyperplasia** can be observed in approximately 50% of newborn babies. **Nappy rash** can occur at any time from birth if skin care is neglected. Parents need to be aware that applying a barrier cream may block the absorbency of modern nappies, allowing urine to sit close to the baby's skin rather than being absorbed into the nappy lining. The excoriated skin is also more vulnerable to *Candida albicans* which should be looked for as both baby and mother (particularly if breastfeeding) may need to be prescribed treatment. By 1 week of age, **seborrhoeic dermatitis** (cradle cap) may also appear but it often occurs later than 2 weeks post birth.

Epstein pearls may be visible as a whitish-yellow, protein-filled cysts on the neonatal gum or palate. A pearl may also be seen on the tip of the penis where it may be mistaken for a blister of more sinister origin. In both cases, these have usually disappeared by the second week of life. A **sucking blister** can often be seen on a baby's hand where it has been suckling in utero. These should be kept clean, but will resolve within a few days.

Atopic dermatitis is a common problem in infancy although it does not usually present until 2–4 months of age. However, if the parents have a family history of eczema, hay fever or asthma, discussing how to reduce possible allergic triggers can have a positive effect on the severity of the condition if it does appear. According to Hormukai (2014), the daily application of an unperfumed moisturiser during the first 8 months of life and using cotton next to the baby's skin can help.

Vascular immaturity

Harlequin colour change is seen most frequently in preterm babies and is thought to be a vascular manifestation of the changes that occur in the autonomic system in the newborn. When a baby lies slightly on its side, this condition presents as a marked paleness along the upper part of the body (Figure 31.1b). It can affect 10% of term babies, usually lasting for a few seconds or minutes, but it is transient and without any other anomalies it requires no treatment. Similarly, **acrocyanosis** is a benign condition that can be seen during the first week of life. It is characterised by bluish hands and feet as the neonatal circulation stabilises after birth. It is unaccompanied by other anomalies and usually resolves by 1 week of age.

Cutis marmorata (marbled skin)

Neonates who have cooled will particularly exhibit this condition whereby the skin, particularly on the legs, demonstrates a marbled effect (Figure 31.1c). Some areas of the skin will be vasodilated (look red), whereas others will be vasoconstricted (look pale) because of the immaturity of the nerves linked to superficial capillaries. Regular assessment of the baby – particularly temperature – should be instigated. At first, re-warming may heighten the colour differences, but gradually the phenomenon will disappear. It should be explored as to why the baby became cold in the first place and if the condition is slow to resolve the baby's blood sugar levels should be evaluated and the possibility of infection (in which physiology requires more energy use) should be explored. There is a permanent form of this condition (congenital generalised phlebectasia), but it is rare and will be exacerbated on crying.

32 Atypical skin conditions

Figure 32.1 Mongolian blue spot.
Source: Lissauer and Avroy (2011). Reproduced with permission of John Wiley & Sons.

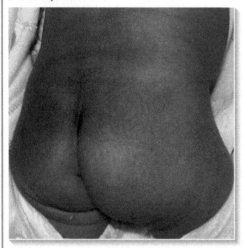

Figure 32.2 Congenital melanocytic naevus.
Source: Lissauer and Avroy (2011). Reproduced with permission of John Wiley & Sons.

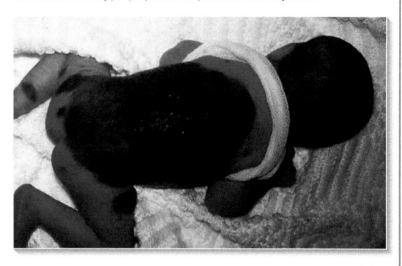

Figure 32.3 Port wine stain.
Source: Lissauer and Avroy (2011). Reproduced with permission of John Wiley & Sons.

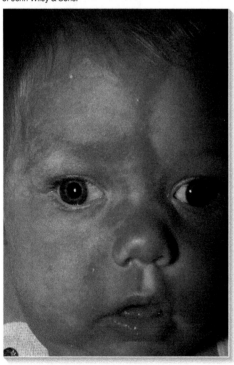

Figure 32.4 Embryonic milk lines.

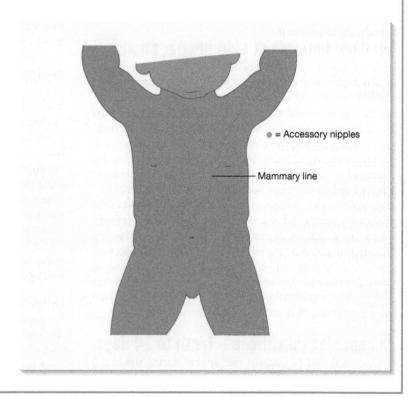

● = Accessory nipples

— Mammary line

Pigmented birthmarks

Congenital dermal melanosis

Congenital dermal melanosis (Mongolian blue spot) presents at birth as faint or well-pigmented blue or blue–grey macules in babies of Asian, African, American, Hispanic, Mediterranean origin or from mixed race conceptions (Figure 32.1). The macules tend to appear over the lower sacrum and buttock, but can also occur on thighs, arms and shoulders. Most will usually gradually fade by 6 years of age, although a few more persistent types may still be visible into adulthood. It is rare for any to appear over the face, head or over the front of the trunk. These require referral, particularly if numerous or presentation appears 'scattered' as there may be a link to other atypical pathologies and forms of potentially serious dermal melanocytosis.

It is paramount that the site, size and shape of these macules are documented, preferably using a body map. This assists in preventing the macules being mistaken for bruising and possible non-accidental injury which could lead to referral to a paediatrician, the involvement of social services and the police, plus being the cause of intense anxiety for the parents.

Sebaceous naevi

These naevi occur in 1 in 300 neonates, either at birth or within the first year. They usually appear as elevated, orange–brown granular plaques on the face and/or scalp which develop uniform, wart-like projections. If any change occurs in appearance, referral will be required for expert opinion (Swetman et al., 2011).

Congenital melanocytic naevus

This naevus develops at birth in approximately 0.3% of neonates. Naevus usually occurs as a brown–black area of the skin which is often flat, but can occasionally be hairy or raised (Figure 32.2). Size must be recorded accurately, as it has been suggested that any naevus measuring greater than 1.5 cm requires referral (Lissauer and Fanaroff, 2011). Some newborns present with multiple naevi or with a 'garment' naevus which covers part of the body and the concern with these latter naevi is the risk of malignancy and therefore expert management is required. Even with smaller naevi, the parents need to know that, as with any mole on the body, any change to the size, texture, thickness or colour will need to be assessed and protection from sunlight is paramount.

Capillary vascular malformations

Naevus simplex

Naevus simplex is the most common mark to present at birth (40%). Dilated superficial capillaries show as poorly defined flat pink macules on the upper eyelid or above the brow line and mid forehead (also known as salmon patch; angel kiss), or in the hair line at the nape of the neck (stork bite). Although the latter may persist into adulthood, the others tend to fade during the first 12 months. However, if this type of birthmark appears elsewhere on the body the baby should be referred for further investigation, particularly if over the spine.

Port wine stain

Port wine stain (naevus flammeus) presents at birth as a flat red or purple patch (Figure 32.3). The cause for this capillary malformation is unknown, but it is more common in girls and occurs in about 0.3% of children (Birthmark Unit, 2012). In time, the lesion thickens, becomes darker and develops an irregular 'cobblestone' appearance. Early referral to a specialist is recommended so that decisions can be made regarding laser treatment or cosmetic camouflage. Laser treatment usually achieves good results and would be considered after the age of 6 months. Port wine naevus in certain areas may carry specific risks (e.g. around the eye) as it increases the risk of glaucoma; around the forehead and scalp it may be associated with fits (Sturge–Weber syndrome), and large lesions on the limbs may be associated with extra growth of the arm or leg (Klippel–Trenaunay syndrome; Birthmark Unit, 2012).

Congenital haemangiomas

These developmental errors of abnormal angiogenesis are the most common benign tumours in childhood. Haemangiomas present in approximately 3% (3 females : 1 male) of the population, with the majority appearing within the first month of life.

Strawberry haemangioma

A benign tumour or birthmark consisting of a dense, often raised cluster of blood vessels in the skin it is a common capillary malformation occurring in 5% of the population. Most become obvious during the first month of life, presenting as a small red patch. They tend to grow rapidly during the first year, after which 90% have usually regressed by approximately 9 years of age. However, some children will be left with scars, telangiectasia or hypopigmentation. It can be difficult to assess how deeply the haemangioma has penetrated the skin. If it interferes with respiration, feeding, hearing, vision, or it ulcerates or bleeds excessively, treatment will be required, often in the form of oral propranolol, steroids or laser treatment. Otherwise, treatment is usually unnecessary and parents are advised to await spontaneous resolution (McLaughlin et al., 2008).

Pre-auricular nodules and sinuses or pits

Unilateral, bilateral or multiple fleshy papules present in the pre-auricular area of the ear, but unless accompanied by any signs of a congenital syndrome are often treated later by cosmetic surgery if wished. Peri-auricular sinuses have a higher occurrence in individuals of Asian or African descent (4%) compared with approximately 0.9% in the Caucasian population. They can occur bilaterally but are more common as unilateral anomalies. The literature is contradictory as to whether they are related to hearing problems (Solak, 2016). However, there is a need to be vigilant for infection within the sinus which if recurrent will need expert excision.

Supernumerary nipples

Accessory mammary tissue can occur anywhere along the embryologic lines (the 'milk-line') that run on each side of the body from the axillae to the inner thighs (Figure 32.4). Accessory nipples can occur anywhere along these lines, but the further away from the breast tissue the less mammary tissue will be present. In neonates, the accessory nipple appears as a tiny, light brown macule. In adulthood, it appears as a small brown papule which protrudes slightly above skin level. In women, if this papule is very close to or on the breast itself and has underlying breast tissue, milk may be produced postnatally.

Neonatal seborrheic dermatitis (cradle cap)

It is thought that this condition occurs as a result of overactive sebaceous glands which are stimulated by the residual maternal hormones in the baby. It appears as a greasy scaling of the scalp which looks a little inflamed. Mild cases will often resolve within a few weeks without needing treatment. Otherwise, the scalp will respond well to being frequently washed with shampoo and gently removing any loose, softened scales. If necessary, an emollient can prove useful, but if the condition continues an antifungal shampoo and/or mild topical corticosteroid can be prescribed (Watkins, 2016).

33 Head

Figure 33.1 Newborn skull showing bones, suture lines and fontanelles.

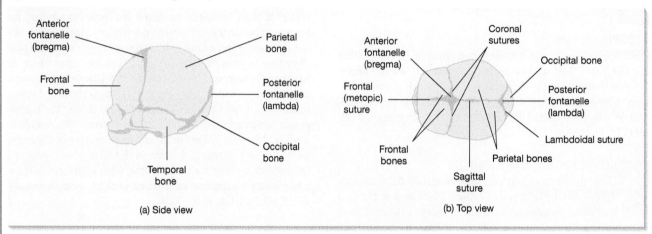

Anterior fontanelle (bregma)

Frontal bone

Parietal bone

Posterior fontanelle (lambda)

Occipital bone

Temporal bone

(a) Side view

Coronal sutures

Anterior fontanelle (bregma)

Frontal (metopic) suture

Occipital bone

Posterior fontanelle (lambda)

Lambdoidal suture

Frontal bones

Parietal bones

Sagittal suture

(b) Top view

Figure 33.2 Measuring the anterior fontanelle.

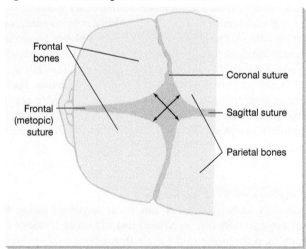

Frontal bones

Coronal suture

Frontal (metopic) suture

Sagittal suture

Parietal bones

Figure 33.3 Caput succedaneum or cephalhaematoma.
Source: Adapted from Brozansky *et al.*, (2012). Reproduced with permission of Elsevier.

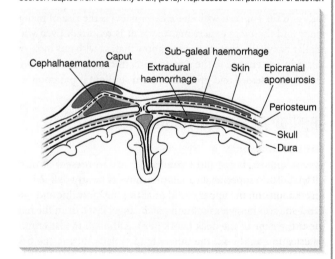

Cephalhaematoma

Caput

Extradural haemorrhage

Sub-galeal haemorrhage

Skin

Epicranial aponeurosis

Periosteum

Skull

Dura

Figure 33.4 Moulding related to positions and presentations.

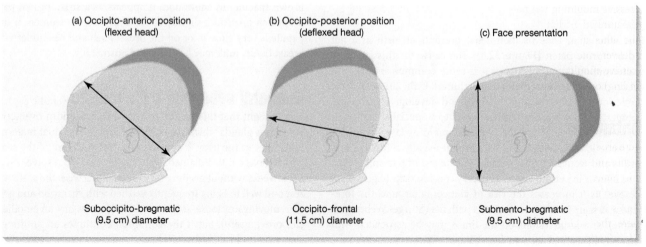

(a) Occipito-anterior position (flexed head)

Suboccipito-bregmatic (9.5 cm) diameter

(b) Occipito-posterior position (deflexed head)

Occipito-frontal (11.5 cm) diameter

(c) Face presentation

Submento-bregmatic (9.5 cm) diameter

This chapter considers the examination of the vault of the skull and scalp, including inspection and palpation of the seven bones, suture lines and fontanelles (Figures 33.1 and 33.2). The practitioner is looking for signs of trauma; excessive moulding; swelling; ridges; decompressions; unusual diameters; bulging or sunken fontanelles; birthmarks; lesions; or abnormal head circumference measurement.

Head circumference

The head circumference (occipito-frontal circumference) indirectly measures the brain, cerebral fluids and skull. At term, for boys this is in the range of 33.1–35.8 cm (15–85th centiles with a 50th centile of 34.5 cm); for girls, 32.7–35.8 cm (15–85th centiles with a 50th centile of 33.9 cm; World Health Organization, 2007). This measurement can be affected by pathological abnormalities but typically will be altered by harmless oedema, moulding or haematoma. Measure the widest diameter to include the occipital and frontal prominences (1–2 cm above the glabella) using a disposable, non-stretchable tape. Take three measurements (to the nearest millimetre) and record the largest of these.

Head shape and moulding

Moulding is a normal process resulting from the movement of the skull bones when compressed before or during labour. The skull bones bend slightly and overlap partially (at suture lines or fontanelles) to reduce the diameters of the head and facilitate delivery. Diameters under pressure reduce by up to 1 cm whilst those without pressure elongate. The degree and direction of moulding relate to fetal positioning and the pressure experienced (Figure 33.4). Moulding is harmless unless it is excessive, rapid or decompresses too rapidly.

The head shape can be significantly affected by fetal presentation antenatally; type of delivery; length of labour; maternal pelvic shape; and by the presentation and position of the fetus during labour and delivery. For example, the breech presentation infant delivered by caesarean section will have a round-shaped head never having experienced any prolonged pressure, whereas the deflexed head of a baby in the occipito-posterior position will experience upward moulding along the submento-bregmatic diameter (Figure 33.4).

Excessive moulding

Excessive moulding is a particular risk for the softer skull of the premature infant. For this to occur in a term infant, there will need to be either an abnormal head or excessive pressure during labour or delivery such as with dystocia or an instrumental delivery. This excessive moulding may damage the bones (through excessive bending) or intracranial membranes, vessels or tissues.

Fontanelles

There are six fontanelles. The two sphenoid and two mastoid fontanelles only show with increased intracranial pressure. The two main fontanelles are the rhomboid or kite-shaped anterior fontanelle (bregma) where the frontal (metopic), coronal and sagittal sutures meet, and the triangular posterior fontanelle (lambda), where the sagittal and lambdoidal sutures meet. Inspection and palpation must be carried out on a quiet, calm newborn as crying will tense the fontanelles. Assess for size, swelling,

decompression, tenseness, bulging or sunken appearance. If unsure, re-examine with the newborn in a sitting position.

The size is measured diagonally, from bone to bone in both directions (Figure 33.2). The two results are added together and divided by two. The bregma is 0.6–3.6 cm (average 2 cm) and can take 6–24 months to close (average 14 months). The lambda is smaller at 0.3–1.5 cm (average 0.6 cm) and typically closes by 2 months. An enlarged bregma (or delayed closure) may be associated with hypothyroidism, achondroplasia (dwarfism), trisomy 21 (Down's syndrome), rickets or increased intracranial pressure. A small bregma can indicate microcephaly. A third fontanelle, between the anterior and posterior fontanelles, may be associated with hypothyroidism and trisomy 21. Bulging fontanelles may be associated with intracranial pressure, hydrocephalus, inflammation (encephalitis), hypoxia, trauma, tumour (scalp or intracranial), heart disease or metabolic disorders. A sunken fontanelle is associated with dehydration.

Common abnormalities

Abrasions or lacerations of the scalp – caused by interventions (amnihook, scalp electrode, fetal blood sampling, instrumental delivery, operative delivery); resolve spontaneously.

Aplasia cutis congenita – typically 1 cm wide, hairless, scalp lesion in front of the lambda. Can be flat, keloid, blistery or ulcerated, with possible exudate. Rarely, associated with an underlying defect – most resolve but leave a bald patch.

Asynclitism – asymmetry of the head resulting from uneven pressure on a tilted head during labour. Resolves spontaneously without problems.

Caput succedaneum (Figure 33.3) – oedema of the presenting part caused by cervical pressure or vacuum extraction. Present from birth. Pits with pressure. Crosses suture lines. Resolves within days.

Cephalhaematoma (Figure 33.3) – blood between the periosteum and bone. Does not cross suture lines, may appear after birth, takes weeks or months to resolve. May cover a fracture.

Craniosynostosis – premature closing or fusing of a suture. Limits growth in the area fused so causes uneven head shape. Associated with rickets, hyperthyroidism and numerous syndromes.

Fracture – usually linear, may be depressed. Rarely, leak cerebrospinal fluid via nose or ear (requires antibiotics). Depressed fractures may require surgery but most fractures heal without problems.

Hair – low hairline, increased quantity, brittleness are more common with congenital abnormalities.

Hydrocephalus – increased cerebrospinal fluid.

Macrocephaly – head circumference above 90th centile.

Microcephaly – head circumference below 10th centile.

Subgaleal (subaponeurotic) haemorrhage (Figure 33.3) – appearance of scalp oedema but contains blood. Present at birth; increases; spreads; resolves over 2–3 weeks. Rare cases lead to massive haemorrhage, shock and death.

Tumour – extracranial or intracranial.

Vascular skin lesions (birthmark) – multiple visible haemangiomas require investigation of possible occurrence on internal organs too.

Whorls – hair follicles slope with skin stretch linked to growth of head. More than two whorls, or any over the parietal region, may be linked to abnormal brain growth.

34 Facies

Figure 34.1 Normal ear position.

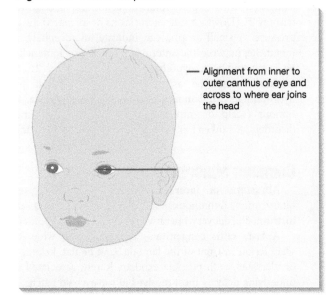

— Alignment from inner to outer canthus of eye and across to where ear joins the head

Figure 34.2 Normal eye position.

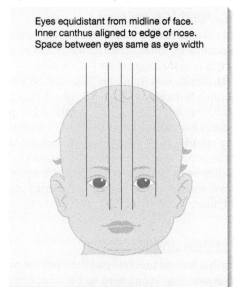

Eyes equidistant from midline of face.
Inner canthus aligned to edge of nose.
Space between eyes same as eye width

Figure 34.3 Normal external ear.

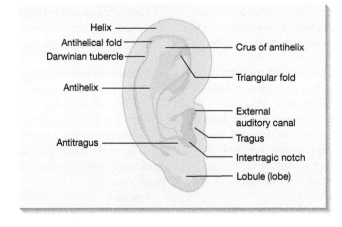

Helix
Antihelical fold
Darwinian tubercle
Antihelix
Antitragus
Crus of antihelix
Triangular fold
External auditory canal
Tragus
Intertragic notch
Lobule (lobe)

Physical Examination of the Newborn at a Glance, First Edition. Denise (Dee) Campbell and Lyn Dolby.
© 2018 John Wiley & Sons, Ltd. Published 2018 by John Wiley & Sons, Ltd.

This chapter considers the facial characteristics, including the nose and extending to the ears. The eyes and mouth have their own more detailed chapters and these should be read in conjunction with this chapter. Whenever possible, it is prudent to consider the facial features of the parents (for familial tendencies) as well as to any relevant history.

Asymmetry and dysmorphia

Assessment of facial symmetry and dysmorphia should take place whilst the newborn is quiet as well as during crying. Look for any lack of uniformity across the two halves of the face; depression of the jaw (micrognathia, may be associated with Pierre Robin syndrome); abnormality in shape, size, structure or positioning of individual features; or the occurrence of any unexpected aspect. The eyes should be the same size and equidistant from the midline of the nose, with the inner aspect of the eyes aligning with the outer width of the nose (Figures 34.1 and 34.2). There should be approximately one eye's distance between the two eyes. Orbital hypotelorism and hypertelorism are the names given to eyes that are too close or too widely spaced apart, respectively. If a problem is identified, an opinion is needed on whether this is a temporary issue (positional pressure in utero or delivery trauma), a deformity or evidence of a syndrome or chromosomal abnormality. Observation during crying aids identification of reduced or absent movements and this includes drooping of the mouth and loss of forehead wrinkles (facial paralysis linked to the 7th cranial nerve).

Skin

The facial skin is inspected for evidence of bruising, trauma, cyanosis, jaundice, birthmarks, tumour or spots. The most common causes of trauma link to the presentation and type of delivery. A face or brow presentation and associated pressure from the cervix or forceps application can cause significant trauma. The degree and placement of any trauma must be documented very accurately to monitor improvements or worsening and to prevent allegations of abuse. Discoloration of the skin and dysmorphia can result from any birthmark but particularly haemangiomas where the tumour develops over or is attached to a facial feature.

The skin colour can also be affected by jaundice and resultant yellowing of the face and sclera. Harlequin syndrome can extend to the face – a phenomenon in which redness, because of increased peripheral blood supply, occurs on one side of the body (often lowermost side) whilst reduced pigmentation and pallor occur on the opposite (and often uppermost) side. Circumoral cyanosis (blue discoloration around the mouth only) may be a normal presentation in the first 24 hours after birth. Similarly, a mild red to purplish coloration during crying can be associated with polycythaemia and this will resolve as the newborn's high haemoglobin level resolves. Any generalised cyanosis, spreading to the body, needs further investigation of full airway patency, pulmonary disease, sepsis or neurological concerns.

Lesions, spots, pustules and blisters occur commonly on the face. These must be identified to inform and reassure parents; advise management as appropriate. The most common are benign erythema toxicum and milia.

Nose

The nose is examined for its appearance, site, symmetry (to the midline), shape, patency, lesions, secretions and for signs of excessive sneezing. There are a wide range of normal shapes but many syndromes can affect the nose. A flattened or low bridge is associated with Down's or fetal alcohol syndrome (FAS) and a short broad nose can be associated with Noonan's syndrome or FAS.

Newborns are nose breathers when at rest but mouth breathers when crying. Hence, cyanosis apparent when the newborn is resting but that clears during crying can indicate nasal blockage. The most common blockage is choanal atresia (see Figure 40.3) which will not be visible but a deviated septum, narrowing or absence of the nostrils, lesions or external malformation of the nose should be looked for. In cases of partial blockage, nasal flare may be evident as a result of greater effort required to nose breathe.

Newborn nasal secretions are minimal and are either clear or slightly frothy (linked to the clearing of amniotic fluid). Yellow secretions occur during pulmonary infection and thick white discharges can indicate viral inflammation. Heavily frothy discharge may be seen with oesophageal atresia. Nasal congestion is rare at birth but may be present by 6 weeks. It is more commonly associated with inflammation and allergy caused by dry air or irritants than infection. Sneezing is generally normal but when excessive can indicate drug withdrawal and neonatal abstinence syndrome.

Philtrum

Long, indistinct, absent or deeper than normal grooves below the nose to the upper lip can be associated with chromosomal abnormalities and syndromes such as Prader–Willi, Noonan's and FAS. Broader than average groves can be seen in those with autism spectrum conditions.

External ear (auricle or pinna)

Ears are examined for shape, site, symmetry (to the face and each other), attachment, lesions and structural abnormality. Patency is covered by the hearing tests but signs of atresia are also assessed. Anotia is the term given to absence of an external ear; microtia is associated with an abnormally small ear (often malformed); and macrotia is an enlarged ear, often otherwise normal but sometimes linked to haemangiomas. The ear should be well formed (Figure 34.3), with the upper margin aligned with the inner and outer canthus of the eye (Figure 34.1). Some initial swelling or squashing of the ear may be positional or a result of delivery but the cartilage should recoil easily to a normal position.

Thickening of the outer or inner aspect of the helix, at the point where the top third begins (Darwinian tubercles, Figure 34.3), are common but rarely significant. Hairy ears may be familial, relate to a syndrome or link to maternal diabetes mellitus. Clefts, grooves, dimples, pits, skin tags, sinuses and fistulae may be abnormalities of aesthetic concern only or may contain cartilage, cysts or tumours and be associated with deafness or a syndrome. Malformed, abnormally attached or low set ears may also link to chromosomal or urogenital abnormality and deafness (e.g. trisomy 17 or 18; Noonan's syndrome).

35 Eyes

Figure 35.1 (a) Common form of coloboma; (b) red eye reflex; (c) congenital cataract.
Source: Lissauer and Fanaroff (2011). Reproduced with permission of John Wiley & Sons.

Coloboma

Cataract

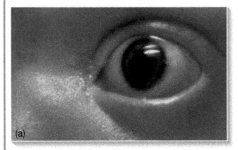
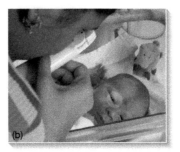
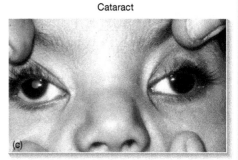

(a)　　(b)　　(c)

Table 35.1 Risk factors for congenital cataract.

Risk factor	Comments
Congenital cataract (*prime risk factor*)	First degree relative Can be inherited as an autosomal dominant condition
Low birth weight	<1500 g
Low gestational age	<32 weeks' gestation May be caused by trauma rather than prematurity per se
Family history of: • Glaucoma • Retinoblastoma	Eye disorder of childhood onset
Maternal infection	Congenital rubella syndrome Toxoplasmosis Cytomegalovirus
Trisomy 21	5–10% of babies will have cataracts at birth Continued reassessment required
Galactosaemia	Caused by changes in the metabolism of carbohydrates and an excess of sugar in the blood and in the aqueous humour disrupting normal development
Idiopathic	50% will have no identifiable cause

Table 35.2 Examination findings.

Screen negative	No anomalies found – make appropriate record within neonatal notes, Personal Child Health Record, NHS Trust digital record and SMART system (if available)
Screen positive	Includes the absence of any reflex – suggesting possible congenital cataract Presence of aleukocoria (white reflex) – suggests a retinoblastoma (a tumour of the eye) Action: • Refer to neonatologist • Assessment with consultant ophthalmologist/paediatric ophthalmology service by 2 **weeks** of age Record, NHS Trust digital record and SMART system (if available)
Screen positive at 6–8 week infant examination	Baby will be referred as above to be seen by 11 **weeks** of age
Information for parents as to when to seek advice (Public Health England, 2016)	• Baby does not open his/her eyes, focus or follow small movements • Baby's eyes look unusual • One eye demonstrates a lack of 'red eye' in a photograph of the baby

Box 35.1 Development of binocular vision.

• Binocular vision requires an unobstructed route for light to enter and reach the back of the eye
• Ongoing development of the motor system must be uninhibited to allow gradual coordination of eye movement
• Requires continual development of the sensory system in order to strengthen the message pathways to the brain, integrating two monocular signals (one from each eye) into one 'binocular' perception

In the UK, approximately 200 children are born each year with a congenital cataract in one or both eyes, but only 40 of these will have a family history of the condition. Cataracts account for the highest (20%) treatable cause of blindness in the UK. Therefore, early detection of congenital conditions such as cataracts is paramount if the child is to achieve the optimum possible visual acuity.

Formation of the eye

Formation of the eye commences at approximately 22 days post conception. By the third trimester, the fetus can detect bright light. At birth, a baby can see objects up to 25 cm away (the approximate distance from the mother's face to the baby whilst feeding). Babies are attracted by highly contrasting patterns of black and white or primary colours. A baby should be able to fixate on an object, with a particular preference for faces, and begin to follow it even when a couple of hours old, although the macula is poorly developed at birth so precise fixation is not possible. However, any ocular condition that interferes with fixation and ocular stimulation can delay or reduce the ability to develop binocular vision (Box 35.1) and social interaction or parental bonding.

Eye examination

Prior to physical examination, the maternity records should always be reviewed for the presence of risk factors (Table 35.1). The parent(s) should also be asked if there is any family history of eye disorders in childhood and the purpose of the examination should be explained. It should be noted if the eyes have been seen since the baby was born as a very small proportion of babies are born without one eye and, even rarer still, an absence of both eyes.

The examination is best carried out when the baby is calm and alert and therefore is often an opportunistic assessment. If the baby is reluctant to open his/her eyes, they should **not** be forced open as trauma can occur to the soft tissue and infection can be introduced. Carrying out the examination in a darkened room, holding the baby over the parent's shoulder or raising and lowering the shoulders of the baby whilst in the supine position may help.

The examination should be undertaken using an 'outwards–in' approach, whereby the outer aspects of the eye are examined first. Size, shape and alignment of the eye(s) should be noted, with the length of one of the baby's eyes corresponding to the distance between the two eyes. The soft tissue surrounding the eye may be oedematous as a result of pressure against the bony pelvis, but this will resolve during the next 24 hours, but drooping of the eyelid should be documented and the baby referred to a paediatrician. Eye lashes should sweep outwards (inward-facing lashes can cause corneal scarring) and there should be no signs of infection. Conjunctivitis presents as a sticky discharge with accompanying redness. The most common causes in neonates are chlamydia, gonococcal or herpes simplex virus infection. A severe and/or untreated infection can lead to scarring of the cornea causing loss of clarity of sight later.

The position, shape, structure and condition of the iris should be noted. A small number of babies have aniridia (absence of the iris or where it has not formed properly) or colobomata. A coloboma (Figure 35.1a) can be recognised by the notch or gap seen within the iris which in itself usually poses no problem for the developing baby (Sinha *et al.*, 2012). However, the malformation of the ocular structure may be more serious and not only affect the underlying structures of the eye, but also the external structures such as the eyelid. It can occur in isolation, but can also appear with other abnormal neonatal features (Sinha *et al.*, 2012).

An ophthalmoscope, using the large, round, white light setting, should be used to shine the light into the baby's eyes from an approximate distance of 30 cm. The ability of the baby to fixate on the light and follow it should be assessed. If there is no obstruction to the passage of light, the beam will bounce off the back of the eyeball toward the front of the eye, eliciting what is termed as the 'red reflex' (Figure 35.1b). The red eye that is sometimes seen in photographs depicts exactly the same response, but the colour may be paler or more creamy coloured with darker skinned babies. However, cataracts, glaucoma and the presence of a retinoblastoma will produce a different response.

Congenital cataract

The early detection of congenital cataracts is the prime reason for conducting the neonatal eye examination. The main risk factor to be noted is a family history of congenital or hereditary cataracts (first degree relative); other additional factors include low birth weight, low gestational age, trisomy 21, family history of any childhood eye disorder and antenatal exposure to viruses (Table 35.1). If the cataract is fully developed, it may be seen (Figure 35.1c) in daylight as a cloudy, silvery disc across the pupil and no red reflex can be elicited when using the ophthalmoscope. Immediate referral to the paediatric team is required with expert referral required within 2 weeks of detection.

Retinoblastoma

This is the most common intraocular tumour to be found in childhood and is a malignant tumour arising from the cells within the retina. Commonly, only a white (leukocoria) reflex can be elicited. Occasionally, later detection may be accompanied by strabismus (squint). The seriousness of this condition should not be underestimated and immediate referral to an ophthalmologist is necessary as the condition can be life-threatening. The emotional impact on the parents is considerable.

Glaucoma

This condition may at first be suspected because of the presence of a watery eye, which may be mistaken for obstruction of the lacrimal duct which drains excess moisture (lubrication) away from the eye. Infantile glaucoma is usually accompanied by a large and cloudy cornea and photophobia. The usual cause is a blockage preventing the drainage of intraocular fluid, leading to a rise in intraocular pressure and enlargement of the globe of the eye with accompanying pressure to the optic nerve. Again, prompt referral to an ophthalmologist is paramount.

Examination findings and documentation

The examination findings should be clearly documented including the actions taken in the event of a screen positive outcome (Table 35.2). As with many aspects of the examination of the newborn, parents will need emotional support in the event of abnormal findings. Sensitively informing the parent(s) of the nature of the findings and prompt referral to the paediatric team is paramount.

Information for parents

Discussion with the parents should not only include the findings of the examination, but should also raise their awareness as to when to contact their midwife, GP or health visitor in the event of future concern (Table 35.2). However, parents are sometimes unaware of their baby's ability to fixate, follow and blink soon after birth or why the immaturity of the eye muscles can produce a normal transitory 'squint' appearance in their baby. Parents should be reminded how far their baby can see; that babies prefer and see in black and white at this age; that they focus intently on an object or person when they are in learning mode and love being talked to – all of which assists their mental development and strengthens their vision.

36 Mouth

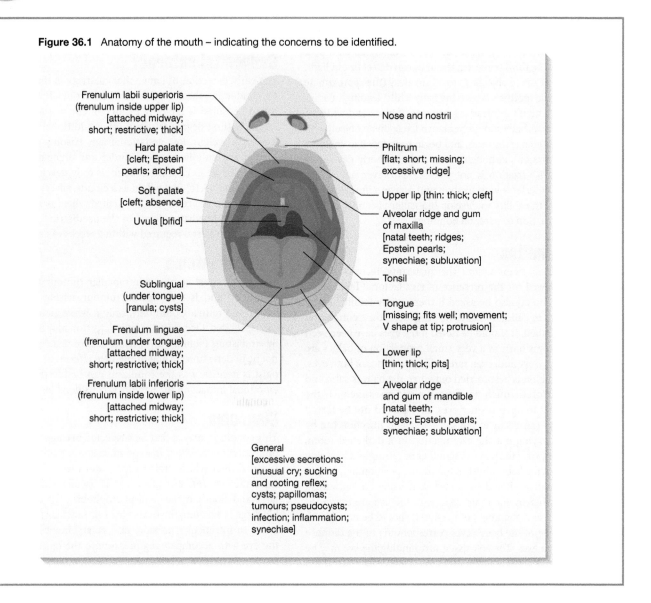

Figure 36.1 Anatomy of the mouth – indicating the concerns to be identified.

Frenulum labii superioris
(frenulum inside upper lip)
[attached midway;
short; restrictive; thick]

Hard palate
[cleft; Epstein
pearls; arched]

Soft palate
[cleft; absence]

Uvula [bifid]

Sublingual
(under tongue)
[ranula; cysts]

Frenulum linguae
(frenulum under tongue)
[attached midway;
short; restrictive; thick]

Frenulum labii inferioris
(frenulum inside lower lip)
[attached midway;
short; restrictive; thick]

Nose and nostril

Philtrum
[flat; short; missing;
excessive ridge]

Upper lip [thin: thick; cleft]

Alveolar ridge and gum
of maxilla
[natal teeth; ridges;
Epstein pearls;
synechiae; subluxation]

Tonsil

Tongue
[missing; fits well; movement;
V shape at tip; protrusion]

Lower lip
[thin; thick; pits]

Alveolar ridge
and gum of mandible
[natal teeth;
ridges; Epstein pearls;
synechiae; subluxation]

General
[excessive secretions:
unusual cry; sucking
and rooting reflex;
cysts; papillomas;
tumours; pseudocysts;
infection; inflammation;
synechiae]

Physical Examination of the Newborn at a Glance, First Edition. Denise (Dee) Campbell and Lyn Dolby.
© 2018 John Wiley & Sons, Ltd. Published 2018 by John Wiley & Sons, Ltd.

This chapter considers examination of the mouth to include the lips, frenulae, palates, tongue, alveolar ridges and gums (Figure 36.1). The mouth is also relevant to the examination of the newborn reflexes (sucking and rooting), feeding and airway management (also see the relevant chapters for these topics).

General congenital abnormalities

Cysts (Scott, 2016) – cavities filled with gas, liquid or a solid mass; oral ones are mostly filled with serous fluid. They are very rare in the newborn but when present can interfere with feeding or swallowing and even occlude the airway. They are typically painless, sterile and less than 2.5 cm in diameter. They can develop anywhere in the mouth and extend into soft tissue, muscle or bone.

Epstein pearls (EP) and Bohn's nodules (BN) – both benign, 1–3 mm wide, cysts. EP are whitish-yellow and found on the gums or roof of the mouth. BN are smooth and white, found either where the hard and soft palate meet or where the gum joins the lip. They disappear naturally by 2–3 weeks of age.

Excessive oral secretions and drooling – occur when a newborn has a poor swallow reflex or in conjunction with oesophageal atresia and tracheoesophageal fistula. Can also appear as a secondary symptom of any condition affecting swallowing (e.g. cysts, tumours and macroglossia).

Pierre Robin syndrome (PRS) – a combination of micrognathia (small mandible) or retrognathia (abnormal position of maxilla or mandible), cleft palate (U-shaped) and a posterior tongue or glossoptosis, which may partially or fully obstruct the airway. Natal teeth may be present.

Subluxation of the jaw – when the upper and lower jaws are not parallel with each other. The lower jaw (mandible) has partially dislocated with one side pushed back. A fetal malposition has resulted in uneven pressure on the jaw, limiting its movement and causing underdeveloped muscles at the hinge joint.

Synechiae (oral) – intermittent adhesions between the lower and upper mouth restricting opening. They may be epithelial or connective tissue alone, or contain muscle and bone. These may be between the:
- mandible and maxilla (syngnathia) – linking the two alveolar ridges;
- tongue and palate (glossopalatal ankylosis);
- floor of the mouth to the palate (subglossopalatal membrane);
- continuous along the alveolar ridges (fibrous syngnathia).

Tumours – granular cell tumours of the anterior maxillary ridge and palate and congenital epulis (gingival cysts of the gums or tongue) are relatively common but they are all benign, occurring mostly in Caucasian but sometimes in Black newborns (Feller *et al.*, 2008).

Lips

- **Thin upper lip** – may be familial but consider fetal alcohol syndrome (FAS) if smooth philtrum and short palpebral fissures seen.
- **Cleft lip** (cheiloschisis) – occurs unilaterally (more common on left side and with male infants), bilaterally or in the midline; in association with cleft palate; may be complete (extending to nose) or incomplete (indentation or grove); and has increased incidence associated with smoking, obesity, diabetes and epilepsy medication (Centers of Disease Control and Prevention, 2015).
- **Enlarged lip** (macroscheilia) – as a result of tumours or partial or complete double lip (horizontal fold and secondary lip).

- **Microstomia** (small width) – often associated with micrognathia.
- **Macrostomia** (large width) – unilateral or bilateral; a transverse cleft extends the side of the mouth across the face.
- **Indentations** – whilst rare, pits, fistulas and sinuses sometimes occur.

Frenula

Each of the frenula should attach midway. They should not appear thick or prominent nor should they abnormally limit movement of anatomy in close proximity. The most common problem identified is tongue tie (ankyloglossia) associated with the frenulum linguae – the tongue tip may be pulled into a V shape with limited extension. Failure to correct the problem through frenuloplasty results in poor latch and nipple pain during breastfeeding, and later speech impediment.

Alveolar ridge and gums

Teeth may be present at birth (natal) or emerge in the first month (neonatal), most commonly lower incisors. Removal is avoided to prevent damage to normal tooth development. If a tooth is mobile (they rarely have firm roots), the risk of trauma or inhalation may necessitate removal. These should be differentiated from EP.

Hard and soft palate, including uvula

Examination must be both digitally and by visualising with a torch.
- **High arched palate** – check for craniostenosis and choanal atresia.
- **Bifid uvula** – associated with cleft palate.
- **Cleft palate** – when the palate at the roof of the mouth fails to fully close during development and a gap (cleft) occurs. It may involve hard and/or soft palate and the alveolar ridge, is more commonly unilateral but can be bilateral and may extend into a cleft lip. Cleft palate alone is more common in girls. It is the most common congenital abnormality (1 : 700 live births): 50% include cleft lip; 15% associated with additional abnormalities (Stringer *et al.*, 2005). In one-third of cases, detection is delayed beyond 24 hours, with increased feeding problems, particularly when either home births or no visualisation (Williams, 2012).

Tongue

Abnormalities of the tongue are commonly associated with metabolic, endocrine or chromosomal abnormalities or tumours.
- **Aglossia** – absence of or poorly developed tongue.
- **Macroglossia** – large tongue protruding beyond the alveolar ridge.
- **Hypoglossia** – short, incompletely developed tongue.
- **Microglossia** – small tongue.
- **Ranula** – translucent, bluish, mucus cyst under the tongue or in the salivary gland; resolves spontaneously.
- **Glossoptosis** – displacement back into pharynx with partial or complete airway obstruction; may be caused by micrognathia (PRS).
- **Dimples, indentations, nodules, grooves and clefts.**
- **Lingual thyroid** – thyroid gland tissue that has incompletely descended and instead enlarges the back of the tongue.
- **Glossitis** – infection may be present (e.g. oral candida [thrush]).

37 Neck and clavicles

Figure 37.1 Webbing and skin folds.

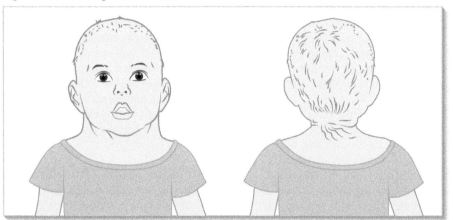

Figure 37.2 X-ray of intact right clavicle.
Source: Image courtesy of Praisaeng at FreeDigitalPhotos.net

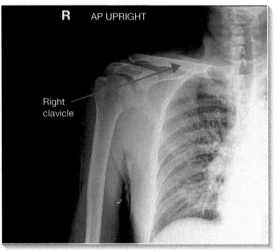

Figure 37.3 X-ray of complete fracture of the left clavicle.
Source: Image courtesy of stockdevil at FreeDigitalPhotos.net.

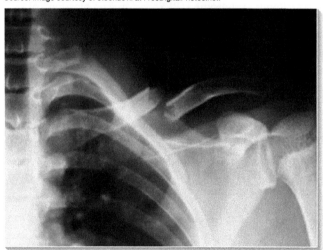

Figure 37.4 Skeleton indicating clavicles.

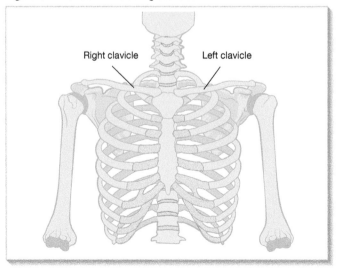

Physical Examination of the Newborn at a Glance, First Edition. Denise (Dee) Campbell and Lyn Dolby.
© 2018 John Wiley & Sons, Ltd. Published 2018 by John Wiley & Sons, Ltd.

Neck

Inspection must include back, front, all creases and up under the chin. This aims to determine the length of the neck, mobility, flexion, symmetry and the presence of any abnormalities. The neck should enable a rotation of the head by 80 degrees to left and right; lateral flexion by 40 degrees; anterior flexion that allows the chin to almost reach the chest; and posterior extension such that the occiput can almost touch the back of the neck. The most common abnormalities detected are the salmon patch (stork mark) and rashes, otherwise the following abnormalities are all very rare and congenital masses are almost always benign. The most important complications to be aware of are the risks to airway and possibility of a syndrome.

Cervical teratoma – rare masses; solid or cystic; typically benign; unilateral; large (up to 12 cm); and likely to cause airway and/or oesophageal compression. Skin is loose over them.

Cystic hygroma – watery tumour associated with lymphatic drainage; relatively rare (1 : 12 000 worldwide) but the most common cervical cystic mass (Ruth, 2007). May occur in the axilla or mediastinum areas too but 90% are cervical and more common on the left. When present after 30 weeks' gestation, it will typically be an isolated condition; before this, a chromosomal abnormality or syndrome is likely, for example, Turner's syndrome, where a short neck and/or neck creases may also be apparent; and trisomies 13, 18 and 21 (Ruth, 2007).

It may require aspiration (decompression) to reduce airway obstruction in the short term. Transillumination can confirm there is no solid mass and magnetic resonance imaging determines the extent of the cyst. Immediate surgical removal is required when the cyst is large, grows rapidly or obstructs the airway; otherwise, it is delayed until the child is approximately 2 years old (Ruth, 2007).

Fistulae or sinuses – rare but occur in skin folds so it is important to visualise the whole neck. First appearance may be of a dimple but examination may determine a deeper fistula or sinus.

Goitre – rare, anterior, midline mass; caused by poor development of thyroid gland and hypothyroidism or maternal medication for hyperthyroidism. Requires hormone replacement therapy.

Haemangioma – these birthmarks mostly occur in the head and neck region.

Rashes – the most common inflammatory condition on the neck is miliaria (heat rash). (Rule out meningitis – ensure no unusual cry, sickness, irritability, floppiness or pyrexia.)

Low posterior hairline – a number of syndromes are associated with hair growth low on the back of the neck (e.g. Turner's, Noonan's and Cornelia de Lange syndromes).

Salmon patch (angel kiss and stork bite/mark) – a common group of birthmarks involving dilated capillaries at the nape of the neck, eyelids and centre of the forehead.

Shortened neck – a number of syndromes are associated with a short neck (e.g. Turner's); with some specifically related to abnormalities of the cervical vertebrae (e.g. Klippel–Feil syndrome). The head should still have full rotation.

Sternomastoid tumour – muscle damage involving painless, benign, swelling within muscle. Can be caused by traction during delivery or intrauterine positioning, affecting blood supply to muscle. Resolves spontaneously but may be associated with a fracture.

Torticollis – restricted movement where a contracted sternomastoid muscle causes the neck to twist or the head to tilt, with chin pointing away from the affected side. It can be related to fetal positioning or instrumental delivery and may be present at birth (congenital) or develop over the first weeks of life. It is painless and corrected by physiotherapy and exercises but can make it harder for the newborn to breastfeed and turn his/her head.

Webbing or excess skin (Figure 37.1) – these are folds that can be extended digitally or taut skin areas. These may also be linked to a syndrome (e.g. Turner's).

Clavicle (collar bone)

The clavicle area should be inspected for shape, distortion and signs of bruising (damaged blood vessels during fracture) (Figures 37.2, 37.3 and 37.4). Clavicles must also be digitally palpated for presence, size, shape, length, callus (spongy lump) and any crepitus. Crepitus will be felt as a grating sensation where the two ends of the fractured bone meet; movement of the bones may even allow crepitus to be heard. The most common abnormality found is a fracture but there are other rare abnormalities such as absence of one or both clavicles (cleidocranial dysostosis) or hypoplasia (congenital pseudoarthrosis).

Fracture

It is very important that vigilant examination takes place in looking for fractures (Figures 37.2, 37.3 and 37.4). Most are incomplete or 'greenstick' fractures and therefore asymptomatic and difficult to detect, but even complete fractures are frequently missed at birth and only identified later when the newborn is more wakeful and demonstrates limited mobility, causing parental concern (Greig, 1999). A birth history of shoulder dystocia, caesarean, ventouse, forceps or extended arms during a breech delivery, or the presence of Erb's palsy post delivery will increase the incidence but fractures are also seen after uneventful spontaneous deliveries. The affected bone will often be the one that was anterior at delivery.

A poor or missing Moro reflex (where the grasp reflex is strong) and asymmetrical movement should arouse suspicion (Greig, 1999). Inspection may elicit an irregularity, depression, bruising, puffiness and crepitus – with signs of pain during the palpation. A callus forms during healing and takes around a week to form so may be present by the 6 week examination. Brachial nerve injury, fracture of the humerus and shoulder dislocation may also be present. Confirmation is by X-ray. Most fractures heal spontaneously but awareness will enable monitoring, analgesia and precautions when caring for the newborn. Care includes loose clothing that opens fully and does not require pulling over the head (to reduce need for movement of affected arm), no lifting from under the arms and securing the arm by pinning the sleeve to the main body of the garment.

Cleidocranial dysostosis

This includes complete or partial absence of one or both clavicles, with the shoulder on the affected side demonstrating unusual ability to bend towards the midline (Tappero, 2009). May be part of a syndrome including multiple skeletal abnormalities and large fontanelles.

Congenital pseudoarthrosis

This is a separated clavicle differentiated from a fracture by the ends each having a smooth, intact cortex without callus formation (Walker et al., 2014).

38 Chest appearance

Figure 38.1 Pectus excacatum (funnel chest) – front view.

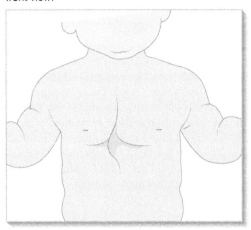

Figure 38.2 Pectus carinatum (pigeon chest).

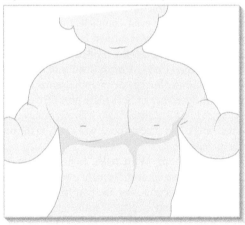

Figure 38.3 AP images of pectus excavatum (top) and pectus carinatum (lower).

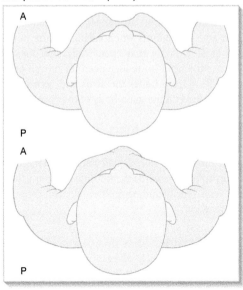

Figure 38.4 Image showing true, false and floating ribs.

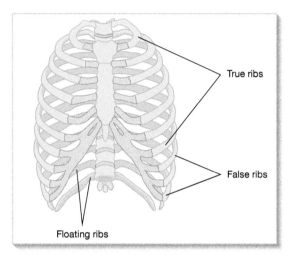

True ribs

False ribs

Floating ribs

Figure 38.5 Most common line of supernumerary nipples (embryonic milk lines).

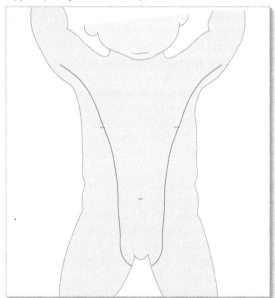

Figure 38.6 Rib abnormalities: bifid, node and notch.

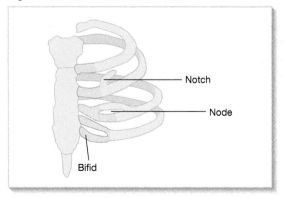

Notch

Node

Bifid

Physical Examination of the Newborn at a Glance, First Edition. Denise (Dee) Campbell and Lyn Dolby.
© 2018 John Wiley & Sons, Ltd. Published 2018 by John Wiley & Sons, Ltd.

Chest examination

This chapter considers the inspection and palpation aspects of the chest. It should be read in conjunction with the other chapters on respiratory assessment. Ideally, it will take place when the newborn is quiet, in a warm environment and with the chest and abdomen exposed, with peripheries covered. This will make the examination easier because the chest and abdomen are relaxed. All relevant history and risk factors should be considered in advance.

Chest inspection

Inspection of the chest area considers the colour, appearance and shape of the chest as well as identification of both normal and abnormal features. There should be no abnormal swellings or depressions (Figures 38.1, 38.2 and 38.3). The skin should be pink with no signs of pallor, cyanosis or enlarged, swollen veins. Any evident rashes or birthmarks should be assessed fully but some rashes such as urticaria neonatorum (erythema toxicum) are normal in the 2- to 5-day-old newborn. Cracking and peeling of the skin is also possible if the newborn was post mature.

The reduced fatty tissue of the newborn and slight intercostal recession may allow some of the ribs to be partially visible against the skin. There are 12 pairs of ribs connected to the vertebra posteriorly. The anterior portions of these ribs are cartilaginous and only the upper 7 pairs are true ribs (reaching the sternum); 8–10 are false ribs (connected to the 7th rib); and 11–12 are floating ribs (not attached to sternum or other ribs; Figure 38.4). Both sides of the chest should be symmetrical and the chest circumference should appear similar or only slightly larger than the abdomen. These should be measured if there is any uncertainty. In a term infant, 31–33 cm is normal or approximately 2 cm smaller than the head circumference.

There should be two nipples evident. In the newborn, these are small pits in the centre of the areola – nipples evert shortly after birth. These will be one on each side of the chest, aligned roughly mid clavicle and at a height just below the axilla. As a result of maternal hormones crossing the placenta in utero, both male and female newborns may have swollen nipples, swollen breasts, lumps under the areola in the breast tissue and there may even be a milky discharge. These conditions are normal and will resolve spontaneously by the 6 week examination. The practitioner should ensure that there is no redness, inflammation, tenderness, pain or any purulent discharge associated with these swellings.

In some newborns, the tip of the xiphisternum will be seen protruding slightly mid chest. This is a small triangular extension of the lower sternum which is still cartilaginous and mobile at birth. It will gradually ossify, become an extension of the sternum and appear less protuberant.

Abnormalities identified on inspection

- **Pectus carinatum** (pigeon chest) – the sternum is pushed outwards into a general V-shaped protrusion at the centre of the chest. It is usually mild and asymptomatic at birth but increases with age.
- **Pectus excavatum** (funnel chest) – the sternum is sunken in the chest causing a visible central depression. This can vary in size but rarely restricts the efficiency of the heart or lungs in a newborn. It may be seen in association with skeletal syndromes (e.g. Marfan's syndrome). Restrictions on lung capacity and pressure on the heart may occur later in life, particularly during exercise.
- **Pneumothorax** – an asymmetrical, enlarged anteroposterior diameter is seen. This can occur spontaneously in an otherwise healthy newborn.
- **Poland syndrome** – under-development of one side of the chest is seen including ribs, muscle and breast tissue. The syndrome can also affect the upper limb on the affected side.
- **Supernumerary nipples** – these are a common minor disorder. Variations occur that include nipples only, areola only, nipples and areola, and some include breast tissue (polymastia). They most commonly occur along the embryonic milk lines (Figure 38.5) but can occur anywhere on the chest and down the abdomen even into the groin.

Chest palpation

Palpation of the chest should ensure that the skin feels warm. The practitioner should feel across the ribs and sternum for evidence of masses, crepitus, thrills or evidence of pain in reaction to touch. It is unlikely that the practitioner will be able to identify increased or decreased numbers of ribs (sometimes associated with trisomy 21), but a severe malalignment or short ribs/short sternum may become evident through reduced chest circumference combined with palpation. If the xiphisternum is protruding then this should be moveable with gentle pressure to ensure it is not a mass.

Abnormalities identified by palpation

- **Abnormal ribs** (fused, bifid, widened or thin ribs; Figure 38.6) – may palpate like a mass on the chest wall, or as reduced or widened intercostal spaces and are associated with a number of conditions including achondroplasia, osteogenesis imperfecta (also associated with fractures), trisomy 18, rickets and hyperparathyroidism.
- **Emphysema** – trapped subcutaneous air that has escaped from the lungs and may be palpated as crepitus. It may result from over-inflation of the lungs (during resuscitation), rib fracture or pneumothorax. Respiratory symptoms of wheezing, tachypnoea and cyanosis will be evident.
- **Fractures** – may palpate as crepitus (crackling/popping feeling) when the two ends of bone rub against each other. Fractures may be associated with resuscitation, difficult delivery or osteogenesis imperfecta.
- **Masses** – chest masses are uncommon but when they occur are more often benign and will have caused rib abnormalities.
- **Thrill** – a vibration that can be palpated through the chest wall; associated with congenital cardiac abnormalities and murmurs.

39 Cardiovascular assessment

Table 39.1 Some of the main family and genetic risk factors for congenital heart defects (CHD).

Risk factor	Likelihood of risk
First degree relative with a history of CHD	Maternal and sibling increases the risk the most from 5% to 10%
Trisomy 12 (Patau)	90%
Trisomy 18 (Edwards)	85%
Trisomy 21 (Down's)	40–50%
Turner's syndrome	35%
Klinefelter's syndrome	15%

Box 39.1 Screen positive findings.

- Tachypnoea at rest
- Episodes of apnoea ≥20 s or associated with colour change
- Intercostal, subcostal, sternal or suprasternal recession, nasal flaring
- Central cyanosis
- Visible pulsations over the precordium, heaves, thrills
- Absent or weak femoral pulses
- Presence of cardiac murmurs and/or extra heart sounds

Table 39.2 Key points of cardiovascular examination.

Observation	General tone	Is the baby floppy?
	Colour (central and peripheral)	Observe colour in daylight, some babies will exhibit 'acrocyanosis' – a normal phenomenon associated with blue hands and feet after birth
	Size and shape of chest	Should be of normal appearance, not barrel shaped, etc.
	Symmetry of chest movement	Movement should be equal on both sides of the baby's chest, there should be no sign of chest recession at the intercostal level (primary) or diaphragm (secondary)
	Respiratory rate	Note rhythm and record rate
	Signs of respiratory distress	No sign of chest recession, nasal flaring or grunting
Palpation	Femoral and brachial pulses	Note strength, rhythm and volume
	Capillary refill time	Depress the nail on the big toe or press gently over the chest – capillary refill time in a neonate should occur within 2 s
	Position of cardiac apex and the presence of thrills	To exclude dextrocardia (heart positioned on the baby's right), obvious presence of cardiac impulse may indicate a heart that is working harder than it should
	Size of liver	To exclude hepatomegaly which is associated with congestive cardiac failure
Auscultation	Presence of murmur?	Determine if systolic or diastolic and if loud or quiet

Table 39.3 Auscultation sites.

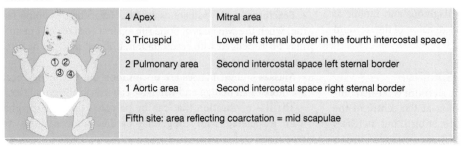

4 Apex	Mitral area
3 Tricuspid	Lower left sternal border in the fourth intercostal space
2 Pulmonary area	Second intercostal space left sternal border
1 Aortic area	Second intercostal space right sternal border
Fifth site: area reflecting coarctation = mid scapulae	

Congenital heart defects

Approximately 1 in 200 babies have a heart anomaly and a comprehensive physical assessment of the neonatal cardiovascular system can assist in the detection of congenital heart defects (CHD). Overall, the incidence of CHD is approximately 4–10 per 1000 live births, ranging from the non-significant to major and critical anomalies. The critical or major congenital anomalies account for approximately 2–3 per 1000 live births. This latter group constitute the leading cause of morbidity and mortality during and after the neonatal period and is further defined by Public Health England (2016a) as:

Physical Examination of the Newborn at a Glance, First Edition. Denise (Dee) Campbell and Lyn Dolby.
© 2018 John Wiley & Sons, Ltd. Published 2018 by John Wiley & Sons, Ltd.

- **Critical CHD** – includes all potentially life-threatening duct dependent conditions and those conditions that require procedures within the first 28 days of life;
- **Major serious CHD** – those defects not classified as critical but require invasive intervention during the first year of life.

Part of the fetal anomaly ultrasound scan encompasses the Fetal Anomaly Screening Programme (FASP) which detects a proportion of critical and major cardiac lesions during pregnancy. However, the 'minimum' acceptable FASP standard detection rate for specific cardiac abnormality is still ≥ 50%. As the neonatal cardiovascular system is still adapting and changing to extrauterine life, a single examination within the first 72 hours of life may not identify all heart anomalies.

Associated risk factors

The key risk factors (PHE, 2016a) for CHD are as follows:

- First degree relative with a history of CHD (Table 39.1);
- Fetal trisomy 21 or other diagnosed trisomy (e.g. trisomy 13 or 18; Table 39.1);
- Cardiac abnormality suspected during antenatal ultrasound;
- Other factors associated with CHD such as maternal rubella, diabetes (type 1), epilepsy, systemic lupus erythematosus and drug-related teratogens (e.g. anti-epileptic and psychotic drugs).

Cardiovascular assessment

It is important that the neonatal cardiovascular examination is comprehensive, detailed and the Newborn and Infant Physical Examination (NIPE) practitioner is highly observant during the examination whilst taking into account if there are any family, antenatal or intrapartum risk factors of relevance.

Parent(s) – prepare and inform

It is also prudent to discuss with the parents if there is any history of CHD within the immediate family as this may not have been noted within the maternal record. The parent(s) should be asked if they have any concerns about their baby's health.

Parents need to be informed that the baby's cardiovascular and respiratory systems are still undergoing changes from intrauterine to extrauterine life. They need to know that as these changes occur it is possible that some murmurs may be heard on auscultation. If the cardiac auscultation is occurring only a few hours after delivery, the parents need to be prepared that hearing cardiac murmurs on auscultation is more likely. Preparation of the parents is important, explaining that sometimes if the baby is fidgety for example, then it may take longer to hear the heart sounds clearly.

Examination process (see Table 39.2 for key points)

Observation

Observation commences at the beginning of the examination and only ends when the practitioner has completed the examination. As the examination progresses, the practitioner should always assess how the baby reacts to increased energy and oxygen requirements as it wakes, moves and interacts with the environment around it. Observe how the baby reacts in response to the examination as it progresses.

Palpation

The practitioner's hand should be placed lightly on the baby's chest in order to ascertain if a 'thrill' or cardiac impulse can be felt through the chest wall – neither of which is normal. Gaining the skill to palpate very small pulse points takes some practitioners longer to master than others. Both brachial and femoral pulses should be palpated and assessed for any discrepancy. The ability to palpate the pedal pulses in the baby's foot can prove useful if palpating the femoral pulse is proving difficult by helping the practitioner to relax and pick up the rhythm of the pulsation.

Link findings relating to the cardiac examination to other parts of the complete examination. For example, finding hepatomegaly (enlarged liver) on abdominal palpation may link to other findings associated with congestive cardiac failure.

Auscultation

Normal heart rate = 100–160/min; respiratory rate = 30–60/min.

Four main sites are used for effective cardiac auscultation (Table 39.3) and a fifth site between the shoulder blades (mid scapulae) can also assist in hearing murmurs that are associated with coarctation. Use an infant-sized stethoscope commencing with the diaphragm (low pitch) the sites 4–1, pause at site 2 and 1 to listen to respiratory air entry and then use the bell (high pitch) to auscultate sites 1–4.

Examination findings

Screen negative

No anomalies found during the cardiovascular examination.

Screen positive

Findings include one or more of the signs and symptoms listed in Box 39.1 that could be suggestive of critical or major congenital heart anomalies (Public Health England, 2016a). Significant murmurs are usually loud, harsh in quality, can be heard over a wide area and are often associated with other abnormal findings. Benign murmurs are typically soft, short, systolic based, localised to the left sternum border and are not associated with other sounds or abnormal findings.

Screen positive findings should always be discussed with a senior paediatrician (neonatologist) or one with expertise in cardiology. The urgency of this consultation will be determined by the clinical condition of the baby. Depending on local Trust policy, initial activity often requires measurement of arterial oxygen saturation (via pulse oximetry) within 4 hours of the examination. However, the Pulse Oximetry Pilot Trial (Public Health England, 2017) has not given the UK NSC conclusive evidence as to whether pulse oximetry screening should be offered across the country. They are at present reviewing the evidence before a final recommendation can be made. Therefore, professionals will need to await this recommendation and follow local Trust policy until a decision is made. However, cardiac anomalies can create life-changing conditions for both the baby and his/her parents. The impact on a parent as a result of a referral for suspected CHD can be profound (Rychik et al., 2013) and referral needs to be expedited smoothly and efficiently, with adequate explanation regarding the reason behind the referral and what will happen and when.

Parental involvement

Parents must always be given comprehensive information relating to the signs and symptoms that they need to be aware of (see Chapter 5), whether their baby is considered to be at risk or not. It is also important to make sure that parents know when to call for an ambulance and the contact numbers for enquiries of a less serious nature.

40 Respiratory assessment and hypoxia

Figure 40.1 Subcostal recession during inspiration.

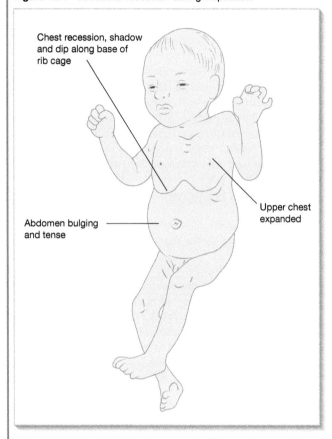

Chest recession, shadow and dip along base of rib cage

Upper chest expanded

Abdomen bulging and tense

Figure 40.2 Intercostal recession during inspiration extending to the sternum.

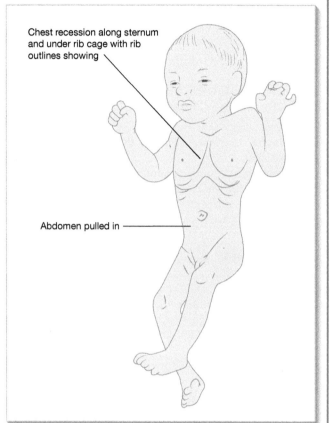

Chest recession along sternum and under rib cage with rib outlines showing

Abdomen pulled in

Figure 40.3 Normal nasal passages showing choanal atresia.

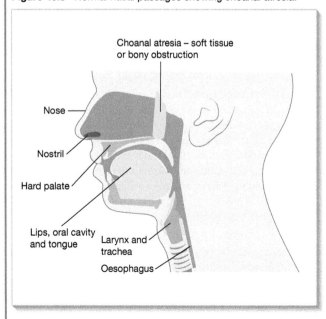

Choanal atresia – soft tissue or bony obstruction

Nose

Nostril

Hard palate

Lips, oral cavity and tongue

Larynx and trachea

Oesophagus

Figure 40.4 Sites of possible congenital airway stenosis from larynx to bronchi.

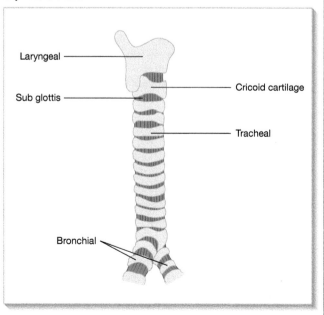

Laryngeal

Sub glottis

Cricoid cartilage

Tracheal

Bronchial

Physical Examination of the Newborn at a Glance, First Edition. Denise (Dee) Campbell and Lyn Dolby.
© 2018 John Wiley & Sons, Ltd. Published 2018 by John Wiley & Sons, Ltd.

Respiratory assessment

Respiratory assessment includes inspection and auscultation of breath sounds. The infant needs to be undressed in a warm environment with peripheries covered to prevent respiratory changes from being cold. As the ribs are still partially cartilaginous and weak, breathing is abdominal and diaphragmatic. As a result, it is the abdomen that can be seen expanding during respiration and the lower thorax may pull in slightly. Nose breathing occurs when babies are quiet but they breathe through the mouth when crying. A normal feeding pattern is reassuring as respiratory problems exacerbate during feeding. Respiratory issues are rarely concealed so should become evident on examination but it should be appreciated that they may be a symptom of problems outside of the respiratory tract (e.g. cardiac anomalies).

Inspection

Inspection should confirm relaxed, symmetrical movement at 30–60 respirations timed over a full minute. The newborn should be a normal pink colour. Peripheral cyanosis of the hands and feet may occur but should not extend centrally, nor to the lips, tongue or mucous membranes. Pallor precedes cyanosis so is also significant. Breathing should not appear to require effort so there should be no nasal flare and any chest recession on inspiration should be very mild and intercostal. It should not extend to the sternum or be deep intercostal or subcostal recession (Figures 40.1 and 40.2). Breathing is generally regular; however, a short episode of erratic breathing and even a 10 s apnoea can be normal. If any irregularity occurs, extend the time observing until reassured; include pulse oximetry and consider chest X-ray.

Auscultation

Auscultation of breath sounds requires a quiet environment and should be via both the bell and diaphragm of the stethoscope. At the initial examination, auscultation routinely occurs subclavicle on both sides of the anterior upper chest. By the 6 week examination, when the chest is larger, routine auscultation occurs in the upper, mid and lower chest cavities on both sides and both anteriorly and posteriorly. Auscultation checks that air entry, inspiration and expiration are all symmetrical and that no abnormal sounds are heard. Sounds are coarser and higher pitched nearer the midline, becoming softer and lower pitched further from the sternum. Secretions, foreign bodies or water will make breathe sounds harder to hear.

Abnormal breath sounds

There are a number of abnormal breath sounds but be aware that breath sounds can be normal even in the presence of conditions as severe as pneumonia. Additionally, whilst abnormality may begin with increased respirations, exhaustion will progress this to slowed respiration and eventual periods of apnoea of 20 s or more. Consider the full picture – breath sounds, respiratory rate (and depth), chest recession and any changes during wakeful periods and feeding. If there is any concern then pulse oximetry is indicated and X-ray may be required.

Apnoea – absence of breathing. Occasional and temporary apnoea (≤10 s) can be normal but may also result from maternal drug use, infection, choanal atresia (Figure 40.3), neurological disease or respiratory distress syndrome.

Bradypnoea – slowed respirations which may also be shallow as a result of traumatic birth (hypoxia or anoxia) or maternal drugs.

Crepitations (crackles or rales) – crackling, clicking or rattling sounds caused by increased lung fluid (e.g. chest infection, pneumonia).

Grunting – expiration through a partially closed glottis. Relatively common and typically resolves spontaneously within 2 hours but may also be associated with infection, hypoglycaemia, hernia and respiratory or cardiac disease.

Rhonchi – low-pitched wheeze, like a snoring sound.

See-saw respirations – extreme chest compression and abdominal bulging on inspiration, with extreme abdominal compression on expiration (e.g. during obstructed airway; Figure 40.4).

Stridor – a harsh vibratory or whistling sound on expiration (e.g. during upper airway obstruction; Figure 40.4).

Tachypnoea – rapid breathing. May be normal before 24 hours (because of retained lung fluid) and resolve spontaneously; otherwise indicates infection, hernia or heart, lung or metabolic disease.

Unequal air entry – may be caused by heart failure, infection, pneumothorax or upper airway obstruction (Figure 40.4).

Wheeze – high or low-pitched whistling sound on expiration caused by inflammation or narrowing of large airways (Figure 40.4).

Hypoxia

This is a condition in which oxygen levels to the brain are reduced. More commonly associated with labour, it can also occur postnatally as an acute or slowly progressing condition when abnormalities of the respiratory, cardiovascular, neurological or metabolic systems occur. Early detection and minimising of damage is essential as damage cannot be repaired.

Choanal atresia

This is the most common nasal airway obstruction and may be unilateral or bilateral (Figure 40.3). Newborns are normally nose breathers when quiet and mouth breathers when crying. If the condition is bilateral, early cyanosis and apnoea is apparent and nose breathing is not possible. In unilateral cases, obstructing the nostrils in turn will help detect which side is affected because obstructing the unaffected side will immediately increase symptoms. Immediate referral is required to enable insertion of an oropharyngeal airway and full investigation of the obstruction.

Pulse oximetry

Pulse oximetry is a screening tool for the measurement of oxygen levels in blood, using sensors placed on the fingers and toes. An air breathing newborn aged 2 hours or more should have a minimum 95% oxygen saturation level. It is used currently when indicated rather than routinely. A pilot carried out by the UK National Screening Committee to consider the feasibility, advantages and disadvantages of routine screening was considered inconclusive because of high false positive reporting and the need for greater understanding of the issues involved (Public Health England, 2017).

41 Upper limbs and hands

Figure 41.1 (a) Normal palmar creases, (b) Oligodactyly (missing fingers), (c) Polydactyly (additional fingers), (d) Single simian crease, (e) Sydney line, (f) Syndactyly (joined fingers).

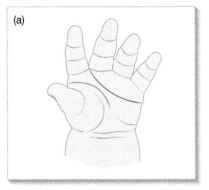
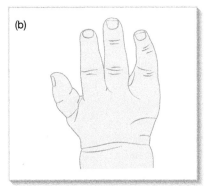
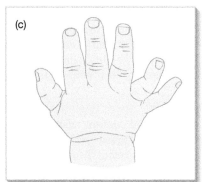
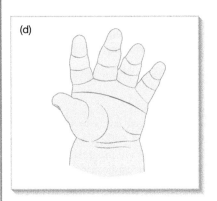
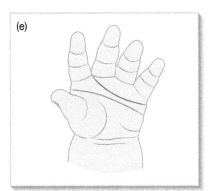
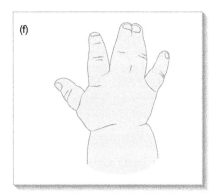

Figure 41.2 Bones of the upper limb and hand.

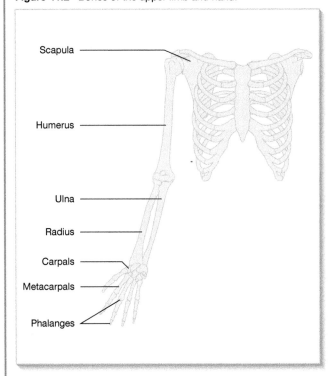

Scapula

Humerus

Ulna

Radius

Carpals

Metacarpals

Phalanges

Figure 41.3 Erb's palsy.

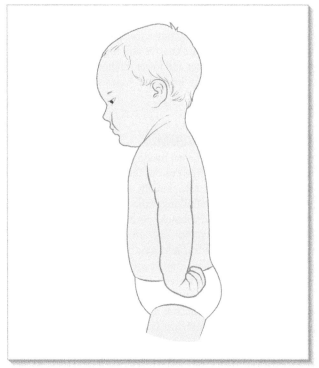

This chapter includes examination of the shoulders, arms and hands (Figures 41.1 and 41.2). Abnormalities of the upper limbs and hands are associated with a range of causes including genetic disorders and syndromes (e.g. achondroplasia and Marfan's syndrome); hypocalcaemia (e.g. hypoparathyroidism); and amniotic bands. Assessment is of bones, joints, muscle and the skin, as well as checking for symmetry of shape and range of movement across the two arms.

Conditions affecting the upper limbs can also affect lower limbs. The best known of these is perhaps the thalidomide birth defects from the late 1950s. A sedative, useful in reducing morning sickness, was bought by 12 000 pregnant women worldwide. For almost half of these, the result was miscarriage or stillbirth. Surviving babies experienced multiple upper and lower limb deformities. Nowadays, the most common causes of upper and lower limb abnormalities are as follow:

• **Achondroplasia (dwarfism) and Kniest dysplasia (disproportionate dwarfism)** – genetic conditions with the production of calcium and collagen reduced; affecting all bone and joint development. Upper limbs will have bowed bones, enlarged joints and short, fat fingers.

• **Radial or ulnar longitudinal deficiency** – a condition that varies in the extent of abnormality. There is poor development and deformities of the upper limbs and particularly the radius and the hands. In severe cases, the lower arms and joints appear significantly curved as a result of short radius, normal ulna and resultant asymmetric growth.

Shoulder abnormalities

When examining the shoulder, the most common injuries to be looked for may be identified by the reduced mobility of the affected arm, absence of reflexes and a birth associated with possible trauma.

Brachial plexus injury – damage to the brachial plexus nerve group through stretching of the nerve roots, which leads to partial or full muscle weakness down the arm and possibly a paralysed arm. Moro and grasp reflexes will be poor or absent and Erb's or Klumpke's palsy may be evident. Spontaneous recovery is common, supported by physiotherapy by the parents, but may take 6 months. If no recovery is evident by this time then surgery may be required and the prognosis for full recovery becomes poor.

Erb's palsy (Figure 41.3) – results from a high brachial plexus injury and is recognised by the 'waiter's tip' positioning. This is when the limp arm rotates inward slightly, with loss of flexion at the elbow and the hand flexes at the wrist to face backwards and upwards.

Klumpke's palsy – results from a low brachial plexus injury and affects the forearm and hand with muscle damage causing a 'clawed hand' shape.

Dislocated shoulders – rare, resulting from direct trauma at birth, brachial plexus injury or as a congenital defect. Dislocations are recognised by internal rotation of the arm, flexion of the wrist and a normal grasp but absent Moro reflex. Movement is limited and asymmetrical with sensation apparent through evidence of pain. The affected shoulder may appear flatter than the unaffected side.

Arms

Examination of the arms inspects for fractures (humerus, radius or ulna), dislocated elbow and abnormalities, with awareness that the elbow will not completely straighten because of a mild flexion contracture (Figure 41.2).

Amniotic constriction band – fibrous bands from the amnion wrap around the developing fetus inhibiting growth, from slight indentations to complete prevention of limb formation.

Dislocated elbow – when the radius and/or the ulna have been pulled out of line from the humerus. It is a very rare birth injury recognised by immobility, pain and malalignment.

Fractures – fractured humerus is the second most common fracture for a newborn after the clavicle. Fractures of the radius or ulna are rare. Indicators are traumatic delivery, caesarean section, restricted movement and pain. It is rarely possible to detect a fracture (unless there is significant malalignment) until a callus forms 7–10 days later.

Limb reduction defects – affects either upper or lower limbs and occasionally upper and lower at the same time.

Tumours – growths that may be deeper within the arm or on the skin (e.g. haemangioma).

Hands and fingers

When examining the hands, each finger and the thumb must be opened fully and inspected along to the nails. The palm, back and sides of the hand must all be checked. Nails can be soft but should be smooth and extend to the finger tips. The normal hand position is in a fist with the thumb tucked in but a persistent fist may be a sign of nerve damage. Techniques to encourage the hand to open include stroking either the back of the hand or the ulnar side. Abnormalities can be individual or part of a syndrome and include the following:

• **Absent or deformed nails** – may be nail–patella syndrome.
• **Arachnodactyly (spider legs)** – long, thin fingers. Associated with connective tissue disorders (e.g. Marfan's syndrome).
• **Brachydactyly** – short fingers.
• **Camptodactyly** – abnormally bent fingers; fixed flexion.
• **Clinodactyly** – a curving finger; may cause overlapping.
• **Kniest dysplasia** – long, knobbly fingers and no fist shape.
• **Macrodactyly** – one or more enlarged fingers.
• **Oligodactyly** – one or more absent digits (Figure 41.1b).
• **Overlapping** – flexed fingers rarely overlap. If the index finger overlaps this can be associated with trisomy 18.
• **Polydactyly** – one or more extra digits (Figure 41.1c).
• **Short, fat digits** – seen in achondroplasia and hypoparathyroidism.
• **Simian crease** (Figure 41.1d) – single palmar crease; commonly associated with trisomy 21 (short finger, incurved little finger and low-set thumb also likely). Occurs with many other genetic conditions and in a small number of unaffected newborns.
• **Sydney line** (Figure 41.1e) – like the simian crease this is associated with trisomy 21 and also congenital rubella.
• **Symbrachdactyly** – short fingers, plus webbing.
• **Syndactyly** (Figure 41.1f) – fused fingers; may be at skin level or include bone.
• **Trident hand deformity** – low attachment of thumb; third and fourth fingers project laterally; associated with achondroplasia.
• **Webbing** – may be reduced (limiting movement) or increased (either extending up the length of the finger or as excessive folds).

42 Abdomen

Figure 42.1 X-ray indicating organs of abdomen.
Source: image courtesy of stockdevil at FreeDigitalPhotos.net.

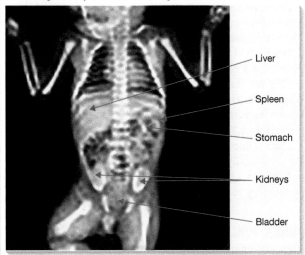

- Liver
- Spleen
- Stomach
- Kidneys
- Bladder

Figure 42.2 Gastroschisis.
Source: Lissauer and Fanaroff (2011). Reproduced with permission of John Wiley & Sons.

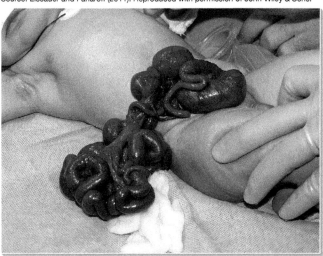

Figure 42.3 Types of oesophageal atresia.
Source: Lissauer and Fanaroff (2011). Reproduced with permission of John Wiley & Sons.

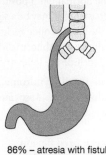 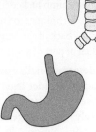 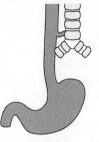

86% – atresia with fistula between distal oesophagus and trachea

8% – atresia without fistula

4% – H-type fistula without atresia

Figure 42.4 Frothy oral secretions linked to oesophageal atresia.
Source: Lissauer and Fanaroff (2011). Reproduced with permission of John Wiley & Sons.

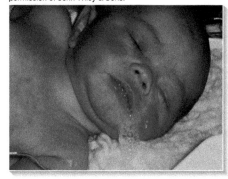

Figure 42.5 Omphalocele.
Source: Lissauer and Fanaroff (2011). Reproduced with permission of John Wiley & Sons.

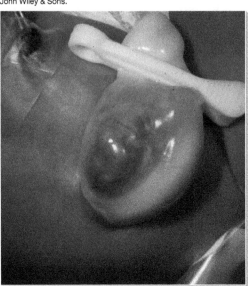

Figure 42.6 Abdominal masses and their causes. Source: Lissauer and Fanaroff (2011). Reproduced with permission of John Wiley & Sons.

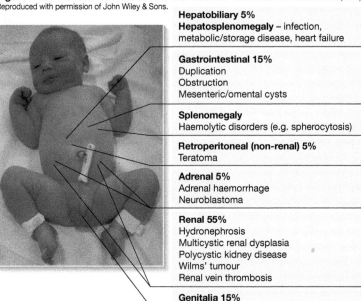

Hepatobiliary 5%
Hepatosplenomegaly – infection, metabolic/storage disease, heart failure

Gastrointestinal 15%
Duplication
Obstruction
Mesenteric/omental cysts

Splenomegaly
Haemolytic disorders (e.g. spherocytosis)

Retroperitoneal (non-renal) 5%
Teratoma

Adrenal 5%
Adrenal haemorrhage
Neuroblastoma

Renal 55%
Hydronephrosis
Multicystic renal dysplasia
Polycystic kidney disease
Wilms' tumour
Renal vein thrombosis

Genitalia 15%

Physical Examination of the Newborn at a Glance, First Edition. Denise (Dee) Campbell and Lyn Dolby.
© 2018 John Wiley & Sons, Ltd. Published 2018 by John Wiley & Sons, Ltd.

Abdominal examination

This chapter considers the inspection and palpation aspects of the abdomen. Ideally, this should take place when the newborn is quiet, in a warm environment, with the chest and abdomen exposed, with peripheries covered. This will make the examination easier because the chest and abdomen are relaxed (Figure 42.1). All relevant history and risk factors should be considered in advance, paying particular attention to ultrasound results regarding any organ abnormalities or polyhydramnios detected (associated with increased risk of oesophageal and duodenal atresia). It will be important to ask about feeding, stools and micturition patterns, as well as inspecting evidence of any vomiting.

Abdominal inspection

Inspection of the abdomen examines for colour, size, shape, symmetry, movement and evidence of any abnormality. The skin should be pink and the abdomen should appear soft and symmetrically rounded, without swelling or depression. The abdominal muscles and skin should appear well toned. Some flattening or distension is possible linked to time of last feed, but the abdominal circumference typically remains between 31 and 34 cm for a term infant. As the newborn is a diaphragmatic breather, it is normal for the abdomen to move more than the chest during respirations.

The umbilical area should be dry, with no offensive odour or discharge. If the examination is on the day of birth then identify the two arteries and one vein. If a single artery is seen or identified at birth, ensure urine has been passed and antenatal ultrasound was normal. Any green discoloration may indicate meconium passed in utero so check the intrapartum history. A clean healthy umbilical stump is dry by the second postnatal day and has separated by 10–12 days.

Abnormalities seen on inspection

Many abnormalities are identified at or shortly after birth, such as gastroschisis (Figure 42.2), bladder exstrophy, ascites, hydrops fetalis, necrotising enterocolitis, malrotation and volvulus. Other abnormalities become obvious once feeding commences or symptoms worsen.

- **Abnormal colour** – duskiness indicates poor circulation or bowel necrosis; redness indicates inflamed bowel.
- **Diaphragmatic hernia** – weakness of diaphragm muscles causes scaphoid (sunken) abdomen; allows organs to push into chest cavity.
- **Diastasis recti** – separated rectus abdominus muscle allows protrusion down the central line of the abdomen particularly during crying; corrects naturally.
- **Duodenal atresia** – a closed part of duodenum; upper abdominal distension; vomiting (even long after feeds); urination and bowel movements stop after first few.
- **Epigastric hernia** – small firm palpable nodule between xiphoid process and umbilicus; fat protruding through muscle weakness.
- **Hirschsprung's disease** – absence of nerve cells regulating colon; affects short or long portion; obstruction, distension, failure to pass meconium and green or brown vomit.
- **Meconium ileus** – distended abdomen and meconium impaction. Most are associated with cystic fibrosis.
- **Oesophageal atresia and tracheoesophageal fistula** (Figures 42.3 and 42.4) – oesophageal obstruction, often with missing portion; commonly with fistula to trachea; distension; frothy oral secretion.
- **Omphalitis** – redness and inflammation of the umbilicus; can track back into the abdomen if not managed early.
- **Omphalocele** (Figure 42.5) – herniation of abdominal contents into the umbilical cord, surrounded by clear sac.
- **Organomegaly** – enlarged organs causing abdominal distension.
- **Prune (wrinkled) belly** – (Figure 38.5) reduced musculature of abdomen.
- **Supernumerary nipples** – may occur on the abdomen.
- **Umbilical granuloma** – excessive granulation causes a red fleshy swelling of the umbilicus; most resolve spontaneously.
- **Umbilical hernia** – weak musculature around the umbilicus; may also allow abdominal contents to protrude.
- **Urachal cyst, sinus or fistula** – clear fluid or urine draining from an opening onto the abdomen between the bladder and the umbilicus.

Palpation of the abdomen

Palpation can confirm concerns following inspection but also checks for masses, organomegaly, tense or relaxed musculature, retained urine or stool, signs of pain or another abnormality. Palpate all four quadrants and centrally. Begin gently, to allow the newborn to become tolerant and not distressed, then deeper palpation will be possible. It is normal to feel some gaseous distension, stool and bladder in the lower quadrants. Upper organs, not entirely covered by the rib cage, can be felt in the upper quadrants.

To palpate, stand to the side of the newborn. Apply the flat, palmar surface of the four fingers and progress in a rolling movement upwards, from the iliac crest to the subcostal margin. Begin in the lower right quadrant. Depress 1–2 cm only and do not lift the fingers completely off because the practitioner may miss palpating an area. The liver will be identified in the upper quadrant, 1–2 cm below the ribs; it has a smooth firm edge and should not feel nodular or hard. Next palpate the left side, the practitioner is unlikely to feel the spleen but, if felt, it must not be more than 1 cm below the ribs. To ensure it is the spleen, feel for a notch in its shape and check it moves with respirations. To feel for the kidneys, place a hand under the infant's back between the false ribs and waist to ballot the kidney forward. Press down on the abdomen with the second hand, lateral to the umbilicus, at a 45 degree angle. Each kidney is about 4–5 cm long and feels like a smooth firm flattened plum. The right kidney is lower and easier to feel. Lastly, feel for a bladder. Begin at the umbilicus and palpate downwards feeling for a fullness rising out of the pelvis. It may be felt 1–4 cm above symphysis pubis but should not be a permanent feature. Typically, urination occurs within the first 12 hours of birth and occurs five times over the first 48 hours of life.

Abnormalities detected on palpation

- **Hepatomegaly** – enlarged liver.
- **Hydronephrosis** – enlarged kidney resulting from fluid. May resolve spontaneously if urine and not a result of malformation, tumours, polycystic kidneys or infection.
- **Masses** (Figure 42.6) – plus any nodules felt on any organ.
- **Pyloric stenosis** – a firm oval shaped mass in the upper mid abdomen; not present at birth but may be felt at 6 weeks.
- **Splenomegaly** – enlarged spleen.
- **Tenderness** – distress and drawing up of knees during palpation may be a pain reaction.

43 Back, spine, buttocks and anus

Figure 43.1 Normal curvature of the spine.
Source: (a) adult image courtesy of rajcreationzs at FreeDigitalPhotos.net.

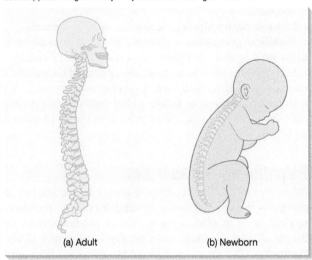

(a) Adult   (b) Newborn

Figure 43.2 X-ray showing spinal scoliosis.
Source: image courtesy of stockdevil at FreeDigitalPhotos.net.

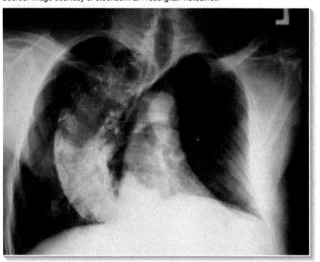

Figure 43.3 Spina bifida occulta, a defect in vertebra – without spinal cord damage, or prolapse of meninges.
Source: Lissauer and Fanaroff (2011). Reproduced with permission of John Wiley & Sons.

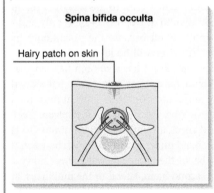

Spina bifida occulta

Hairy patch on skin

Figure 43.4 Meningocele, a defect in vertebra with prolapse of meninges – without spinal cord damage.
Source: Lissauer and Fanaroff (2011). Reproduced with permission of John Wiley & Sons.

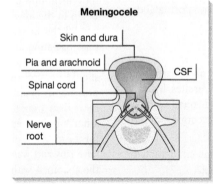

Meningocele

Skin and dura
Pia and arachnoid
Spinal cord
CSF
Nerve root

Figure 43.5 Myelomeningocele, a defect in vertebra and skin – with prolapse of meninges and spinal cord.
Source: Lissauer and Fanaroff (2011). Reproduced with permission of John Wiley & Sons.

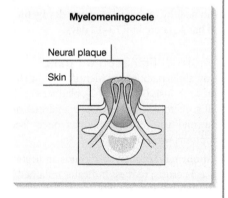

Myelomeningocele

Neural plaque
Skin

Figure 43.6 Myelomeningocele.
Source: Lissauer and Fanaroff (2011). Reproduced with permission of John Wiley & Sons.

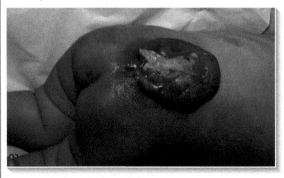

Figure 43.7 Occipital encephalocele.
Source: Lissauer and Fanaroff (2011). Reproduced with permission of John Wiley & Sons.

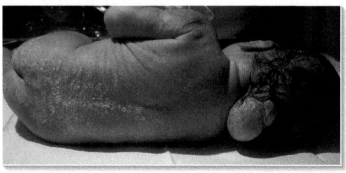

Physical Examination of the Newborn at a Glance, First Edition. Denise (Dee) Campbell and Lyn Dolby.
© 2018 John Wiley & Sons, Ltd. Published 2018 by John Wiley & Sons, Ltd.

The examination begins with awareness of the history for any risk factors, paying particular attention to anomaly screening (e.g. nuccal space; banana or lemon sign; sibling history; anticonvulsant therapy; alpha-fetoprotein [AFP]). Reassuring factors include antenatal folic acid therapy and normal head and neck (see Chapters 33 and 37). Antenatal management makes it unlikely that major abnormalities will remain undetected. However, not all women accept screening and false negatives can occur (e.g. skin-covered spinal lesions will not raise AFP levels). Signs that are not detected antenatally will be the less obvious ones, making care during this examination even more important.

Working in a light, warm environment, lie the newborn prone over the hand and lower forearm. Inspect for changes in normal skin colour, hairy patches (other than lanugo), deformity, dimples (of any depth), masses and evidence of a normally situated patent anus. Visualising the passage of stool will be a reassuring feature (see Chapter 27). Palpation covers the whole back and full length of the spine, ensuring normal curvature and that all spinal processes are felt.

Back

The back is examined for any abnormalities of the skin, curvature and scapulae. The back of a newborn baby does not have changes in curvature. The prone position, lying over the forearm, should enable confirmation that the back is convex (Figure 43.1). The skin should have no birthmarks or evidence of masses. It is covered in inconspicuous fine hairs but may also have noticeable downy unpigmented hair (lanugo) for a few weeks. Dark hairs may be seen on Asian babies – wider cuticles make the hair more noticeable. Excessive hair may relate to hormone imbalance and requires investigation. The scapulae (shoulder bones) should be roughly triangular in shape, with a flat surface. The upper border is roughly horizontal, below clavicle height and with normal shoulder movement.

Congenital dermal melanocytosis (Mongolian blue spot) – occurs in single or multiple patches. Document their presence to ensure they are not mistaken for bruising and abuse but they are not associated with underlying concerns.

Sprengel's deformity – small, winged or raised scapulae with the lower point protruding; typically unilateral, making the scapulae asymmetrical. A raised effect may make the neck appear webbed and limits movement. Check for scoliosis and Klippel–Feil syndrome.

Spine

Examine from the base of the skull to the coccyx, looking and feeling for changes to the skin colour or texture; tufts of hair; soft or cystic masses; dimples; cysts; or sinus tracts. The most common congenital spinal deformities are associated with abnormal or incomplete development or postural deformities.

Spinal curvature

Congenital spinal curvature may be secondary to in utero positioning or associated with abnormally fused vertebrae. Sitting the infant resting over one hand will sometimes make kyphosis or lordosis more apparent and holding under the arms and raising the infant may make a scoliosis more obvious (Figure 43.2).

Early detection allows corrective management before growth exaggerates the problem. The three main curvatures are:

1 **Kyphosis** – exaggerated curvature of thoracic and sacral regions;
2 **Lordosis** – exaggerated curvature of lower lumbar region;
3 **Scoliosis** – sideways curvature of the spine to left or right.

Spinal neural tube disorders

Spina bifida cystica (SBC) and spina bifida occulta (SBO) are the two main disorders but an encephalocele may occur at the top of the spine where the skull and spine meet (Figures 43.3, 43.4, 43.5, 43.6 and 43.7). Concerns arise if a lump, dimple, hairy patch or naevus are seen over the midline and require further investigation.

Spina bifida cystica – incomplete closure of one or more vertebrae with varying degrees of protrusion of the cord and meninges. Most are lumbosacral.

• *Meningocele* – protrusion of meninges with normal underlying spinal cord; can be dura or skin covered.

• *Myelomeningocele* – protrusion of meninges and spinal cord; most in a sealed sac of cerebrospinal fluid (CSF); flat or bulging. Check for CSF leakage, hydrocephalus, orthopaedic or neurological abnormalities (lower limb paralysis).

• *Myeloschisis* – a myelomeningocele where a mass of nerve tissue has flattened along the skin surface.

Spina bifida occulta – incomplete closure of one or more vertebrae; often asymptomatic as cord is intact; risks increase depending on the size of the defect and number of vertebrae affected. More extensive are associated with a dimple, sinus, hair tuft, naevus or fatty swelling (lipomyelomeningocele).

Spinal or dermal dimple – commonly an innocent sacrococcygeal dimple, particularly if it lies over the coccyx. It could also indicate an underlying spinal abnormality – SBO or a tethered spinal cord. A tethered cord can be stretched and damaged as the infant grows.

Spinal or dermal sinus – a tract down from the skin; may reach the spinal cord but most end in a cyst or tumour. Can occur anywhere but most are lumbar. Observe for leaking CSF. Do not probe as this may introduce infection or cause further damage. May be associated with tethered cord.

Buttocks

The most common abnormalities seen are congenital dermal melanocytosis and sacral dimples but other forms of naevus are possible. A pilonidal dimple is one based above the buttock cleft. Sacral dimples are mostly shallow enough for the base to be seen and are innocent. If it is not possible to see the base then investigate for possible sinus or fistula.

Anus

Examine for position, patency and to ensure that there is no associated fistulae. Patency can only be confirmed by witnessing the passage of stool. Evidence of stool in the nappy is reassuring but not confirmation that it was passed from the anus. Examine dimples to ensure they do not leak stool – a patent anus does not prohibit leakage of stool from a secondary site. Elicit the anal wink reflex (puckering contraction during gentle stimuli) to confirm normal sensory and motor responses and ensure the stool type, quantity and frequency are all normal (see Chapter 27).

44 Developmental dysplasia of the hips

Table 44.1 Observation and manipulation.

Observe for	Screen positive findings are in red	
Normal leg movement when nappy is removed	Does the baby kick, knees abduct naturally, is one leg held in an unnatural position?	
Symmetry of leg length	The practitioner needs to stand at the baby's feet, ensuring that the baby lies straight	Difference in leg length
Level of knees when hips and knees are both flexed	Galeazzi or Allis's sign can be used on babies but not older children or adults as it may prove ineffective	Knees at different levels when hips and knees are bilaterally flexed
Symmetry of skin folds – buttocks and posterior thighs	When baby held in ventral suspension. This symmetry may be questionable in the event of bi-lateral hip dislocation	Asymmetry of skin folds
Manipulation		
Ortolani	Screens for a dislocated hip	
Barlow	Screens for a dislocatable hip. This manoeuvre does not actively seek to dislocate the hip but correct positioning of the femur/femoral head allows detection of instability and in some cases demonstrates dislocation	
Screen positive finding: difficulty during Ortolani to abduct knee to 90 degrees (Public Health England, 2016a) A palpable 'clunk' when undertaking either Ortolani's or Barlow's manoeuvres		

Table 44.2 Ortolani's and Barlow's manoeuvres.

Baby should be lying on a firm, flat surface, straight, relaxed and free from the nappy or surrounding clothing/bedding. The practitioner should stand at the end of the cot

For both Ortolani's and Barlow's manoeuvres
Both legs should be gently flexed to a right angle – the legs should not be over- or under-flexed. This is the neutral position from which both manoeuvres commence and finish. In neonates each hip should be examined separately, not together as this raises the effectiveness of the examination

Ortolani *Side being tested*	*Side not being tested*
Place middle finger on the greater trochanter (outer bony prominence near the neck of the femur) with the thumb round the distal, medial femur In a male baby, take care not to catch the scrotal sac	The hand on this side of the baby is used to stabilise the pelvis preventing sideways roll as the manoeuvre is performed The hand is applied to the baby in a similar fashion as on the side being tested, but the fingers are slipped under the buttock to hold the pelvis and prevent movement
Applying a slight upward pressure to the greater trochanter, the practitioner's hand should rotate the leg/hip outwards until the back of the hand connects with the mattress. The leg should then be returned, in a controlled movement, to its original position	If the baby is fidgety or wishes to kick, the fingers can be placed under the buttocks with the thumb placed firmly, but gently on the symphysis pubis
A *positive sign* is indicated by a palpable 'clunk', jerk or grating as the hip is abducted and returned to the neutral position	Practitioners who are learning can inadvertently exert more pressure on the symphysis pubis than a more experienced practitioner, thus the handhold above is more preferential at first
Barlow *Side being tested*	*Side not being tested*
With the hand in the starting position for Ortolani, the knee should be adducted to the midline and pressure applied down the femur – a backward–downward motion. The adducted angle of the femur should be maintained until the pressure is released and the leg returned to the neutral position	Stabilisation of the pelvis is not so important in preventing the pelvis rolling, but rather it holds the pelvis steady allowing the examining hand to feel the movement of the hip being tested However, the knee/leg on the side not being tested should be allowed to abduct slightly in order to give room for the other leg to be adducted. This helps to initiate an effective adduction and to maintain the angle during the manoeuvre
The manoeuvre is not used to make the hip dislocate but to place it in a position where it might do so if unstable. In this case, the femoral head may move too easily to the brim of the acetabulum (demonstrating laxity/subluxation) or may be pushed posteriorly out of the acetabulum and dislocated – *a positive sign*	

Figure 44.1 (a) Barlow manoeuvre and (b) Ortolani manoeuvre. Source: Figure from Lissauer and Fanaroff (2011). Reproduced with permission of John Wiley & Sons.

(a) Barlow's manoeuvre **(b) Ortolani's manoeuvre**

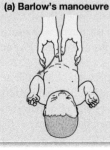
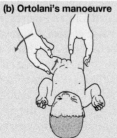

(a) Test for dislocatable hip. The hip is held flexed and adducted to the midline. The femoral head is pushed downwards. If dislocatable, the femoral head will be pushed posteriorly out of the acetabulum
(b) Test for dislocated hip. Abduct hip with upward leverage of femur. A dislocated hip will return with a palpable **clunk** into the acetabulum

Physical Examination of the Newborn at a Glance, First Edition. Denise (Dee) Campbell and Lyn Dolby.
© 2018 John Wiley & Sons, Ltd. Published 2018 by John Wiley & Sons, Ltd.

Developmental dysplasia of the hip (DDH) develops when an abnormal development occurs between the femoral head and the acetabulum of the pelvis. More specifically, DDH encompasses a spectrum of conditions ranging from minor acetabular dysplasia and laxity to irreducible dislocation of the femoral head. Godley (2013) suggested that 1 in 100 babies' hips may be lax or subluxable. Therefore, assessing hip stability is a primary focus of the examination.

The term 'developmental' reflects that this condition can develop any time between uterine life and into early childhood. Hip dysplasia is sometimes referred to as a 'silent' condition as it does not cause pain in babies. Therefore, some cases may be seen presenting late in the neonatal period. It also does not necessarily prevent babies from learning to walk at a normal age. However, DDH can have long-term sequelae such as impaired mobility and pain or osteoarthritis of the hip and back if it remains undetected or when treatment is delayed (International Hip Dysplasia Institute, 2016). Therefore, early detection, diagnosis and treatment can improve later health and reduces the need for surgical intervention. Neonatal instability of the hip is also complicated by its natural history of resolution, in that 60% of dislocatable hips will resolve, with 70–90% resolving spontaneously (Rosendahl *et al.,* 2010).

Predisposing risk factors

In general, the key risk factors for DDH can be identified within the maternal and neonatal records. However, parents should always be asked if they have any concerns or any further information that may be useful. The risk factors identified by Public Health England (2016a) are as follow:

- **First degree relative** – either parent or sibling of the baby that has a history of hip problems as a baby and needed treatment either physically or surgically should be considered at risk of DDH.
- **Breech presentation** – ≥ 36 weeks' gestation, irrespective of the presentation at the time of delivery or the mode of delivery. However, the risk is also higher for any baby delivered earlier than 36 weeks in the breech position. Good observational skills can also detect those babies that have not been detected as lying in the breech position, for example, a baby who has been lying in a frank breech position will often assume a position post birth where the legs are lifted into the air.
- **Multiple birth** – if any baby presented as breech then his/her siblings should also be considered at risk of DDH. NIPE states the rationale that it may be difficult to identify at birth which baby was affected. However, some local NHS policies will investigate further all babies born of multiple conception because of the restricted ability to move easily in a crowded environment.

Raposch *et al.* (2014) and Mace and Paton (2015) also cite the significance and the higher incidence of DDH in female babies.

Examination process

The hip examination is comprised of two parts: *observation* and *manipulation* (Table 44.1). Observation commences from the moment that the legs are visualised. Manipulation consists of both Ortolani's and Barlow's manoeuvres: Ortolani's manoeuvre is used to screen for a *dislocated* hip and Barlow's is used to screen for a *dislocatable* hip.

Only a practitioner experienced in conducting the hip examination should perform it, unless they are observing someone who is training to do so. Both manoeuvres are screening tools only and the more experienced the practitioner, the easier and more effective the manoeuvres.

The baby should be relatively relaxed and examined in a warm environment. Sometimes the assistance of a parent to allow the baby to suckle on a finger during the manoeuvres is required. The parent(s) should be informed that the manoeuvres used do not hurt the baby as they are naturally occurring movements. However, the baby may become irritated because of his/her legs being held and because often this manoeuvre occurs at the end of the examination process.

The baby should be lying on a firm, flat surface (the maternal bed flexes too much) which will assist in the effectiveness of Ortolani's and Barlow's manoeuvres used to assess hip stability (see Table 44.2 for an explanation of how these manoeuvres are performed).

The examination findings should be documented within the neonatal record, digital record and SMART system (if available) and in the Personal Child Health Record. Any anomalies must be discussed with the neonatologist and the practitioner should be aware of local policy regarding referral (see Tables 44.1 and 44.2 regarding screen positive findings).

Examination findings

Screen negative examination, no risk factors

No anomalies found during the examination and no risk factors have been identified so no further action is required.

Screen negative examination, with risk factors

Refer for hip ultrasound within 6 weeks. Babies with no predisposing risk factors but are found to have 'clicky' hip (high-pitched click – usually ligamentous in origin) should be managed as per the local referral policy as they are not included in the NIPE Screening Programme key performance data.

Screen positive

One or more of the screen positive factors (Public Health England, 2016a) indicates the need for the baby to be referred to the neonatologist and undergo hip ultrasound within **2 weeks.**

A baby found to be **screen positive** following the 6–8 week infant examination will be referred directly to an orthopaedic surgeon for urgent expert opinion which should occur by 10 weeks of age.

Parental awareness

Parents need to be informed to observe their child's leg movement and if they have any concerns to contact their midwife, GP or health visitor. In particular, Public Health England (2016a) advocates that parents should observe for the following:

- A difference in the deep skin creases of the thighs between the two legs;
- One leg cannot be moved out sideways as far as the other when changing the baby's nappy;
- One leg seems to be longer than the other;
- A click can be felt or heard in one or both hips;
- One leg drags when their baby starts crawling;
- Their child walks with a limp or has a 'waddling' gait.

Natural development of the hips is facilitated by practices that mimic the fetal flexed position, allowing plenty of hip movement, flexion and adduction (Clarke, 2013). Conversely, an unhealthy position, when the legs are held in extension with the hips and knees straight and/or when the legs are brought together (Torjesen, 2013) inhibits hip development, raising the potential for misalignment and dislocation. Therefore, the importance of slings that promote flexion of the hip, car seats with a wide seat base allowing the legs to sit naturally apart and the baby not sitting in a car seat too long should also be discussed with the parents.

45 Genitalia – female

Figure 45.1 Normal female genitalia of newborn.

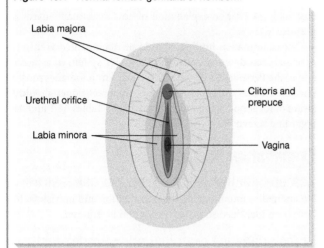

- Labia majora
- Clitoris and prepuce
- Urethral orifice
- Labia minora
- Vagina

Figure 45.2 Inguinal hernia.

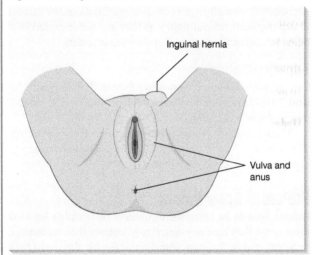

- Inguinal hernia
- Vulva and anus

Figure 45.3 Fusion of labia majora.

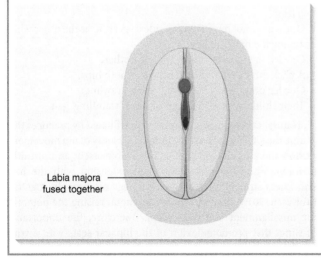

- Labia majora fused together

Figure 45.4 Pseudomenstruation (blood stained, mucus discharge).

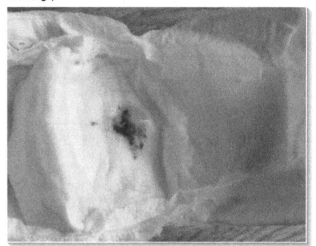

Figure 45.5 Urates – brick coloured, powdery deposits.

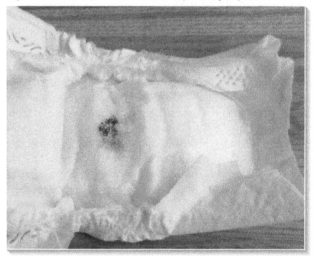

Figure 45.6 Ambiguous genitalia.

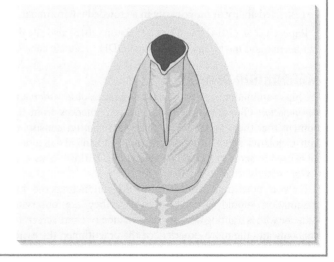

Physical Examination of the Newborn at a Glance, First Edition. Denise (Dee) Campbell and Lyn Dolby.
© 2018 John Wiley & Sons, Ltd. Published 2018 by John Wiley & Sons, Ltd.

Female genitalia

The examination should take place in a warm environment with the groin and genitalia area clean and fully exposed. Inspection includes assessment of the groin, labia, clitoris, vagina, urethra and perineum (Figure 45.1). Palpation confirms the absence of any masses. Earlier palpation of a normal bladder and confirmation of urine output are reassuring features. Appearance of anuria or oliguria up to 48 hours in an otherwise healthy infant may not be a concern if there is no palpable bladder – plus micturition may have been missed. Apply a urine collection bag and a tissue over the urethra to monitor. Risk factors from the full history are important, particularly ultrasound results. Cardiac anomalies, reduced numbers of umbilical cord vessels, oligo- or polyhydramnios and musculoskeletal abnormalities increase the risk of renal and genital anomalies.

Groin

The groin should be flat, without inflammation or swelling, even during crying (when intra-abdominal pressure increases). The femoral pulse should be palpable but not visible, except in a premature or significantly small for dates infant. The most common abnormalities can both occur at the same time.

Inguinal hernia (Figure 45.2) – bulging within the groin area is the most common hernia of the newborn. Incomplete closure of the processus vaginalis allows protrusion of uterus, fallopian tubes or intestines into the soft tissue and labia. The condition may be present at birth but more commonly develops in the first few weeks and should be soft, disappearing spontaneously during rest or able to be digitally reduced and returned to abdominal cavity. Intestine permanently trapped is said to be 'incarcerated'. Enlargement, darkening and hardening of the swelling, accompanied by increasing pain and vomiting, may indicate strangulation (reduction of blood supply and tissue death).

Hydrocele – bulging fluid-filled mass caused by peritoneal fluid within processus vaginalis.

Labia

The labia majora are a normal skin colour and cover the labia minora at term. There should be no skin tags, adhesions or fusion between the two sides of the labia. The skin should not be tense and shiny or be covered in rugae. Some swelling is possible because of the effect of maternal hormones (lasts weeks) or trauma during breech birth (lasts days) and may be accompanied by bruising. The size should not appear disproportionately large or change along the length of each labia. Enlargement, rugae or sack-like swelling arouses suspicion of ambiguous genitalia and indeterminate sex. Similarly, any masses need investigation as they could be one or more testes (ovaries do not descend), a mucoid cyst or, more rarely, a tumour.

The practitioner should gently separate the labia majora to inspect the labia minora. These are usually smaller, brighter pink–red and appear moist. It is also likely that they will be covered in a cheesy white substance. This is vernix which will be naturally absorbed over the first days of life. The most common abnormalities seen are as follow.

- **Adhesions** – can be seen in otherwise normal infants.
- **Fusion** (Figure 45.3) – may be adrenogenital syndrome or ambiguous genitalia.
- **Pigmentation** – increases with ambiguous genitalia and strangulation of hernia.

Clitoris

The clitoris and prepuce (a shorter foreskin) are very prominent at birth (**cliteromegaly**) because of increased circulating hormones including increased androgen production. They protrude from the upper join of the labia minora. The most common abnormality is **bifid clitoris** – a split clitoris, often with no prepuce.

Vagina and urethra

The urethra lies directly below the clitoris but is rarely visible in the newborn unless there is an associated prolapse or cyst. Normal urine streams and a non-palpable bladder are reassuring features. The vaginal orifice should be easily visible below the clitoris, 1.5 cm in diameter and embedded between the pairs of labia. A white mucoid blood-stained loss, associated with maternal hormones, may be evident (pseudomenstruation; Figure 45.4). The most common abnormalities are as follow.

- **Epispadias** – the urethra lies above or to the side of the clitoris; commonly associated with absent or bifid clitoris.
- **Hydrocolpos** – obstruction (possibly imperforate hymen) of vagina with distension because of secretion build-up behind the obstruction.
- **Hydrometrocolpos** – hydrocolpos extended to the uterine cavity.
- **Hymenal tag** – thickened vascular membrane protruding from the vagina with central orifice; common but resolves spontaneously.
- **Imperforate hymen** – hymen has no meatus. Bulges from vagina after obstructing vagina and build-up of secretions.
- **Urates** (Figure 45.5) – combination of calcium and urate crystals, formed during mild dehydration; passed in urine as a brown–pink stain.
- **Urethral polyp** – interlabial protrusion with meatus that leaks urine; rarely obstructs in females.
- **Urogenital sinus/fistula** – dip or channel between urethra and uterus or vagina.
- **Vaginal skin tag** – benign skin growth around vaginal orifice.

Perineum

Examine the perineum for dimpling, fistulas, skin tags, cysts, masses and to ensure that the anus is at least one fingertip away from the genitalia.

Ambiguous genitalia

Ambiguous genitalia include some or all of the following: clitoral enlargement that looks phallic; fusion of labia majora; abnormally located urethral meatus; and/or a palpable mass (Figure 45.6). Increased virilisation (masculinisation) will have occurred. The cause for a female infant will be congenital adrenal hyperplasia – when XX females develop masculinised (androgynous) genitalia following excessive production of testosterone. However, at birth, the female status is not known and the infant should be referred to as 'baby' until the gender can be decided upon. This decision will require involvement of the paediatrician, endocrinologist, geneticist and urologist. They will consider the genetic sex (chromosomal karyotype); gonadal sex (presence or absence of testes); functional sex (possibilities with current organs); and screen for adrenal hyperplasia (ACTH, urea and electrolytes). If a mass is palpated this may be testes as ovaries never descend into or below the groin.

46 Genitalia – male

Figure 46.1 Embryology of testicular descent.
Source: Lissauer and Fanaroff (2011). Reproduced with permission of John Wiley & Sons.

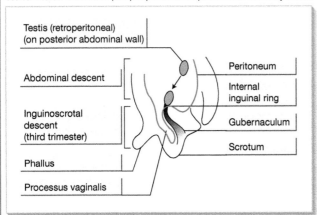

Figure 46.2 Normal obliterated processus vaginalis.
Source: Lissauer and Fanaroff (2011). Reproduced with permission of John Wiley & Sons.

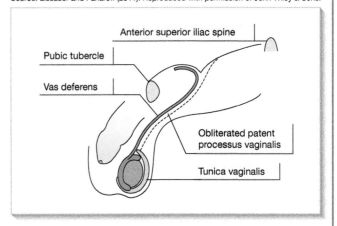

Figure 46.3 Inguinal hernia (widely patent processus vaginalis).
Source: Lissauer and Fanaroff (2011). Reproduced with permission of John Wiley & Sons.

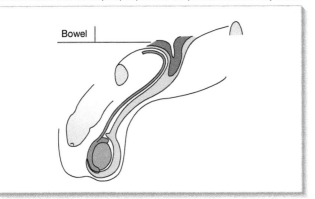

Figure 46.4 Hydrocele (narrowly patent processus vaginalis).
Source: Lissauer and Fanaroff (2011). Reproduced with permission of John Wiley & Sons.

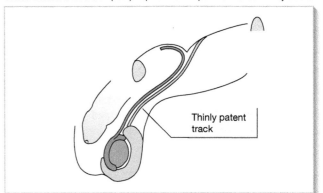

Note: (Fig. 46.1) Embryology of testicular descent. The testis migrates from the posterior abdominal wall to the scrotum. It is preceded by a tongue of peritoneum, the processus vaginalis. This is obliterated in the normal infant (Fig. 46.2). It remains widely patent in an inguinal hernia (Fig. 46.3). With a hydrocele, it is patent but narrow (Fig. 46.4). Source: Lissauer and Fanaroff (2011). Reproduced with permission of John Wiley & Sons.

Figure 46.5 Hypospadias.
Source: Lissauer and Fanaroff (2011). Reproduced with permission of John Wiley & Sons.

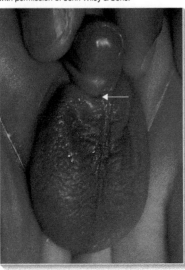

Figure 46.6 Classifications of hypospadias.
Source: Lissauer and Fanaroff (2011). Reproduced with permission of John Wiley & Sons.

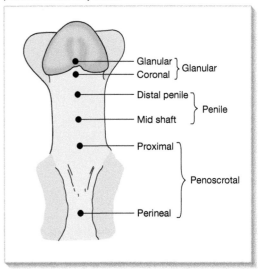

Physical Examination of the Newborn at a Glance, First Edition. Denise (Dee) Campbell and Lyn Dolby.
© 2018 John Wiley & Sons, Ltd. Published 2018 by John Wiley & Sons, Ltd.

Male genitalia

The examination should take place in a warm environment with genitalia clean and exposed. Inspection is of the groin, penis, scrotal sac and perineum. Palpation confirms the presence (or absence) of the testes and assesses for any masses. Earlier palpation of a normal bladder and confirmation of urine output are reassuring features. Anuria or oliguria (up to 48 hours) in an otherwise healthy infant may not be a concern if there is no palpable bladder as micturition may have been missed. Apply a urine collection bag and a tissue over the urethra to monitor. Risk factors from the full history are considered, particularly ultrasound results. Cardiac anomalies, numbers of umbilical cord vessels, oligohydramnios or polyhydramnios and musculoskeletal abnormalities increase the risk of renal and genital anomalies.

Groin

The groin should not appear enflamed or swollen along the line of testicular descent (Figures 46.1 and 46.2) and not bulge even during crying (when intra-abdominal pressure increases). The femoral pulse should be palpable but not visible, except in a premature or significantly small for dates infant.

Inguinal hernia (Figure 46.3) – seen as bulging within the groin area. This is the most common abnormality within the groin. Incomplete closure of the inguinal canal allows protrusion of intestines towards or into the scrotum. It may be present at birth but more often develops in the first weeks. It should be soft, disappearing spontaneously during rest or able to be digitally returned to the abdominal cavity. Intestine permanently trapped is said to be 'incarcerated'. Enlargement, darkening and hardening of the swelling, accompanied by increasing pain and vomiting may indicate strangulation (reduction of blood supply and tissue death).

Penis

The penis should be straight and of normal skin tone. Stretching to 3.5 cm from the pubic bone to the prepuce (foreskin) and glans and 1 cm wide mid shaft; pads of fat over the symphysis pubis can make it appear shorter (micropenis). The prepuce covers the head of the penis. It is not retractable (phimosis) for 2 years but should not be tight. The urethral meatus is a small orifice, typically visible centrally at the tip of the penis, allowing a straight, continuous urine flow. If the meatus is not visible but urine is passed from below the prepuce without it ballooning, this is reassuring – check there is no meatus visible elsewhere. The most common abnormalities of the penis are as follow.

• **Aphallia** – no penis.
• **Bifid penis** – two halves to penile shaft with one urethra; associated with cloacal extrophy (exposure of abdominal organs and bladder).
• **Chordee** – over-developed fibrous tissue with traction and bend of the penis. Downward chordee can be associated with hypospadias.
• **Diphallia** – duplicated penis; bifid or true duplication.
• **Epispadias** – urethral meatus on upper aspect; extremely rare but may be as extreme as bladder exstrophy.
• **Hooded prepuce** – prepuce is absent on the underside of the glans. Common alongside hypospadias.
• **Hypospadias** (Figures 46.5 and 46.6) – abnormal location of urethral meatus under penis, with incomplete urethra. Three types: (i) *glanular* (coronal or balanic) – at base of glans; may include hooded prepuce, shallow pit over end of penis, meatus at lower end of pit; (ii) *penile* (distal or midshaft) – between glans and scrotum; (iii) *penoscrotal* (proximal and perineal) – opens where penis and scrotum join or on the perineum.
• **Micropenis** – short and/or thin penis; beware ambiguous genitalia.
• **Posterior urethral valves** – congenital blockage within the urethra.
• **Priapism** – erections are normal and common.

Scrotum and testes

The scrotum should be symmetrical, slightly darker than surrounding skin, covered in rugae, with a mid-line ridge. The testis are ovoid, firm, smooth and equal in size (1–1.5 cm). When palpating, resist the temptation to press directly on to the scrotum as this can ballot the testes up along the inguinal canal. Instead, begin at the upper groin and, using two fingers, digitally palpate each side, down along the inguinal canal and into the scrotum until the testis is felt (or you are confident it is not within the scrotal sac). All abnormalities must be identified and referred within 72 hours of birth (Public Health England, 2016a,b).

The common abnormalities are as follow:

• **Anorchia** – absence of both testes; must be reviewed by consultant paediatrician or associate specialist within 24 hours (PHE, 2016b).
• **Bifid scrotum** – two separated scrotal sacs.
• **Bruising** – trauma; may be caused by breech presentation or delivery.
• **Cryptorchidism** – unilateral or bilateral undescended testes. If asymptomatic and unilateral, review at 6 and 22 weeks. Bilateral must be reviewed by consultant paediatrician or associate specialist within 24 hours (PHE, 2016b); even when asymptomatic – surgery by 1 year old.
• **Ectopic testis** – starts to descend but stops, often at inguinal pouch.
• **Hydrocele** (Figure 46.4) – fluid-filled scrotum.
• **Oedema** – as a result of hormones or trauma.
• **Pigmentation** – darkening of scrotum; may be a sign of congenital adrenal hyperplasia or torsion of the testes.
• **Smooth scrotum** – associated with anorchia and prematurity.
• **Testicular torsion** – twisted testes; reddened/darkened, swollen scrotum; does not transilluminate; leads to ischaemia and necrosis.
• **Webbed penis** – scrotal sack extends up penis and may reach glans.

Perineum

Confirm there is no additional meatus, fistula or mass and that normal spacing occurs between scrotum and anus.

Ambiguous genitalia

Ambiguous genitalia may result from the following.

• **Undervirilised male** – aphallia; micropenis; smooth scrotum; anorchia or ectopic testes; abnormally located urethra.
• **Virilised female** – cliteromegaly; labial fusion.
• **Ovotesticular disorder** – testicular and ovarian tissue present.

The infant should be referred to as 'baby' until gender is confirmed. This will require involvement of the paediatrician, endocrinologist, geneticist and urologist. They will consider the genetic sex (chromosomal karyotype); gonadal sex (presence or absence of testes); functional sex (possibilities with current organs); and screen for adrenal hyperplasia (ACTH, urea and electrolytes).

47 Lower limbs and feet

Figure 47.1 Anteriorly bowed and flexed legs.
Source: image courtesy of Honza Soukup on Flickr https://www.flickr.com/search/?text=hearing%20test&license=4%2C5%2C9%2C10.

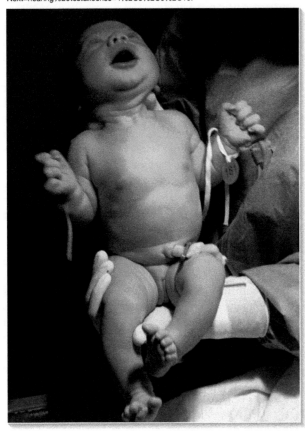

Figure 47.2 Positive Allis' sign with unequal knee heights.

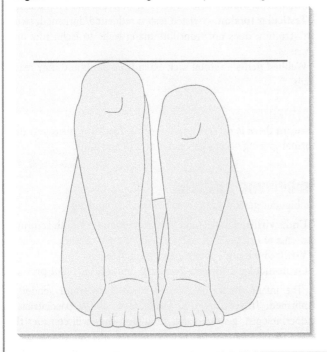

Figure 47.3 Congenital talipes varus.

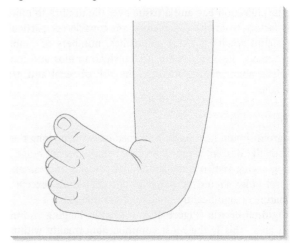

Figure 47.4 Normal creases.
Source: image courtesy of kangshutters at FreeDigitalPhotos.net.

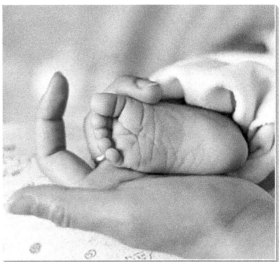

Figure 47.5 Deep plantar crease and wider space between toes (trisomy 21).

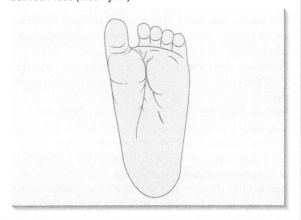

This chapter considers the legs and feet. Assessment of the hip and the reflexes are considered in their own chapters and include assessment of gluteal leg folds. Similar to the upper limbs, abnormalities of the lower limbs and feet are mostly associated with a range of causes including genetic disorders and their resultant syndromes (e.g. achondroplasia and Marfan's syndrome), hypocalcaemia (e.g. hypoparathyroidism) and amniotic bands. Assessment is of bones, joints and muscle and includes checking for symmetry of shape and range of movement across both legs.

Some conditions affect both the upper and lower limbs. Since 1962 and the withdrawal of thalidomide for pregnant women (see Chapter 41), the most common cause of multiple limb abnormalities, which can affect upper as well as lower limbs, is dwarfism.

Achondroplasia (dwarfism) and Kniest dysplasia (disproportionate dwarfism) – involve reduced calcium and collagen, affecting all bone and joint development. The femur is shortened and bowed, joints are enlarged and the toes are short and fat.

Legs

The examination of the legs considers the femur, tibia, fibula, patella, soft tissue and musculature. The practitioner needs to be aware that the legs of a newborn will always appear slightly anteriorly bowed and flexed when at rest (Figure 47.1). Symmetry of the length of the legs should be assessed using Allis' sign (Figure 47.2). This involves the lower legs being bent, feet placed flat and equidistant from the midline, then observing the height of the knees to ensure symmetry – unequal heights are a positive Allis' sign. Rare abnormalities include the following.

Amniotic bands – affect either upper or lower limbs and occasionally upper and lower at the same time.

Congenital femoral deficiency – very rare; associated with shortening or absence of one or both femurs; may extend to tibias, fibulas and the patellae.

Dislocated knee – various degrees of extension of the knee are seen; requiring manipulation to stabilise. Often found in association with developmental dysplasia of the hip and talipes.

Dislocated patella – the patella has moved laterally and the injury is often missed; may occur with trisomy 21.

Fractures – rare but should be considered following a traumatic birth, particularly breech extraction. Shape may be asymmetrical; mobility reduced; painful; irregularities along the bone; bruising or haematoma; crepitus; and a callus forming 7–10 days after delivery. Crepitus will be felt (and may be heard) as a grating sensation where the two ends of the fractured bone meet. However, lower limb fractures are more likely to be avulsion fractures, caused when a ligament or muscle is over-stretched during traumatic delivery and as a result snaps away a small part of the epiphysis.

Limb reduction defects – affect either upper or lower limbs and occasionally upper and lower at the same time. This is when part of, or the whole of a limb fails to develop fully.

Nail–patella syndrome – on examination, the nails are absent or poorly formed and there is an indentation rather than curvature over the knee. The knees may turn inwards and movement is limited; assessment may reveal small or missing patellae.

Sirenomelia (mermaid syndrome) – extremely rare; affecting the spine, pelvis, lower limbs, genitals and lower abdomen (plus internal organs). Newborn has full or partial fusion of the legs. Foot abnormalities include no feet, one foot or backwards-facing feet.

Tumours – very rare; may be deeper within the leg or on the skin (e.g. haemangioma). Any unusual lump or swelling should be investigated.

Feet and ankles

The most common mild abnormality related to the feet and ankles is positional talipes. This is when one or both feet turn inwards (invert). It results from constriction in utero and reduced joint movement. Gentle pressure on the outer side of the soles of the feet enables normal positioning without any discomfort for the newborn.

Talipes – forms of congenital talipes that cannot be gently reduced, affect one or both feet and may combine two types in one deformity:

- *Talipes calcaneus* – when the foot pulls up towards the shin at the ankle (dorsiflexion);
- *Talipes cavus* – a high-arched foot;
- *Talipes equinus* – the foot angles away from the shin at the ankle and points downwards;
- *Talipes valgus* – the foot is abducted and everted; twisted outwards;
- *Talipes varus* (Figure 47.3) – the foot is adducted and inverted; twisted inwards.

Rocker-bottom feet – the heel (calcaneus) is prominent and the talus (ankle bone) has developed further along the foot creating a convex sole. This abnormality is associated with many neuromuscular and chromosomal abnormalities (e.g. trisomy 18).

Simian crease (Figures 47.4 and 47.5) – deeply grooved plantar crease running longitudinally from between the big toe and second toe. Commonly associated with trisomy 21 but occurs with many other genetic conditions and also in a small number of unaffected newborns.

Toes

Many of the abnormalities of the toes are similar to those of the fingers:

- **Absent or deformed nails** – may also have nail–patella syndrome.
- **Arachnodactyly (spider legs)** – unusually long toes. Associated with connective tissue disorders (e.g. Marfan's syndrome).
- **Brachydactyly** – short toes.
- **Camptodactyly** – one or more abnormally bent toes; fixed flexion.
- **Clinodactyly** – a curving toe; may cause overlapping.
- **Macrodactyly** – one or more enlarged toes.
- **Oligodactyly** – one or more absent toes.
- **Polydactyly** – one or more extra toes.
- **Sandal gap** – wide space between first and big toe (trisomy 21).
- **Short, fat toes** – seen in achondroplasia and hypoparathyroidism.
- **Symbrachdactyly** – short toes, plus webbing.
- **Syndactyly** – fused toes; may be at skin level or include bone.
- **Webbing** – this may be reduced (limiting movement) or increased (either extending up the length of the toe or as excessive folds).

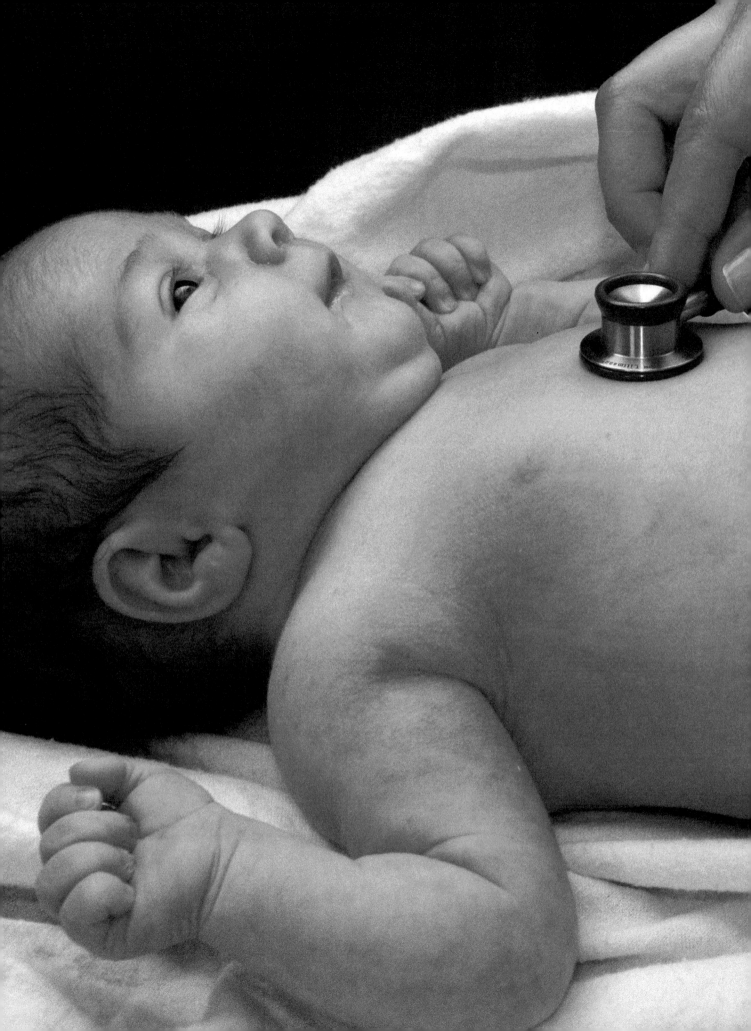

Revision and self-assessment

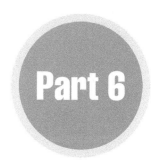

Part 6

Chapters

Section 16 Revision

48 Syndromes and signs

Achondroplasia (dwarfism)

Megalocephaly
Prominent forehead
Protruding jaw
Flat area between eyes
Short limbs
Kyphosis
Lordosis
Associated with – hydrocephalus, upper airway obstruction

Beckwith–Weidemann

Macrosomia
Asymmetrical growth
Macroglossia
Ear creases or pits
Associated with – omphalocele, hernias, hypoglycaemia, enlarged abdominal organs, cancerous and non-cancerous tumour (Wilms' tumour)

CHARGE

C = Coloboma (hole/defect of eye)
H = Heart defects
A = Atresia choanae
R = Restricted growth/development
G = Genitourinary abnormalities
E = Ear abnormalities

Cornelia de Lange

Low birth weight/slow growth
Microcephaly
Excessive body hair
Thin, arched, joined eyebrows
Low-set ears
Long eyelashes
Narrow down-turned lips
Upturned nose
(Mild forms have no signs)
Associated with – cleft palate, gastrointestinal problems, seizures, heart defects, eye problems

Cri du chat

High-pitched, cat-like cry
Hypotonia
Low birth weight/slow growth
Microcephaly
Downward slant to wide-set eyes
Epicanthic folds
Low-set ears
Abnormally shaped/folding ears
Micrognathia
Single palmar crease
Associated with – inguinal hernia, diastasis recti

Crouzon

Early fusion of sutures/fontanelles/facial bones
Brachycephaly
Wide-set, bulging eyes
Strabismus
Beak-like nose
Flattened cheeks
Protruding chin
Low-set ears
Under-developed upper jaw
Concave face
Short humerus and femur
Associated with – narrow ear canal, heart defects, cleft lip/palate

Down's (trisomy 21)

Hypotonia
Flat occiput
Third fontanelle
Upward slanting eyes
Epicanthic folds
Low-set ears
Simple pinna
Short neck
Single palmar crease (simian line)
Short little finger
Wide space between first and second toes
Associated with – omphalocele, duodenal atresia, heart disease, Hirschsprung's disease

Edwards (trisomy 18)

Low birth weight
High mortality rate
Microcephaly
Micrognathia
Small mouth
Low-set ears
Long overlapping fingers
Under-developed thumbs
Clenched fists
Smooth 'rocker-bottom' feet
Kyphosis
Associated with – cleft lip and palate, cardiac and kidney disease, hernias, exomphalos, bone abnormalities, urinary infections

Fetal alcohol syndrome (FAS)

Low birth weight
Reduced head circumference
Small eye openings
Epicanthal folds
Short palpebral fissure
Flat mid-face
Minor ear abnormalities
Short nose
Thin upper lip
Indistinct philtrum
Micrognathia
Associated with – slow growth rate, movement and coordination problems, liver and kidney disease, cardiac disease, hearing and visual problems.

Goldenhar (oculo-auricular-vertebral; OAV)

Incomplete development of eyes, ears, nose, soft palate, lip and mandible – small, missing parts, skin tags, strabismus
Hemifacial macrosomia
Fused or missing vertebra
Scoliosis
Associated with – deafness, blindness, heart defects, limbal dermoids (eye tumours)

Klippel–Feil

Fusion of 2+ cervical vertebrae
Limited neck movement
Shorter neck
Low hairline
Elevated scapulae (Sprengel deformity)
Scoliosis
Asymmetrical limb lengths
Associated with – heart, lung, kidney, genitourinary deformities, cleft palate, spina bifida

Physical Examination of the Newborn at a Glance, First Edition. Denise (Dee) Campbell and Lyn Dolby.
© 2018 John Wiley & Sons, Ltd. Published 2018 by John Wiley & Sons, Ltd.

Marfan

Connective tissue disorder
Longer limbs and fingers
Scoliosis
High palate
Long, narrow face
*Associated with – heart, bones, joints,
lung, eyes, skin and blood vessel
disorders*

Mermaid (sirenomelia)

Legs fused together
*Associated with – kidney, bladder, bowel
and genitalia abnormalities; typically
mortality within 48 hours*

Nail–patella

Affects nails, bones, kidneys, eyes
Small, poorly developed nails
Patellar aplasia – absent, small or
luxated
Elbows misshaped
Scoliosis
Cervical ribs present
Abnormal scapulae

Neonatal abstinence

Amount and type of alcohol/
drug withdrawal
Low birth weight, poor weight
gain
Mottled colouring
Hypertonic
Hyperactive reflexes
High-pitched, frequent crying
Loose stool
Vomiting
Fever
Irritability, jitteriness, seizures
Excessive suck but poor feeder
Sweating
*Associated with – maternal alcohol or
drug dependence*

Noonan

Large head compared with face
Tall forehead
Epicanthal folds
Downward slant palpebral fissure
Short, broad nose
Deep philtrum
Full lips
Micrognathia
Low-set, thickened ears
Posteriorly rotated, oval ears
Oedema of hands and feet
Webbed neck – excess nuchal
skin
Sunken sternum
Associated with – heart defects

Patau (trisomy 13)

Low birth weight
Hypotelorism or cyclops
Cleft lip and palate
Small eyes
Malformed nose
Neural tube defects
Microcephaly
Ear malformations
Polydactyly
Rocker-bottom feet
*Associated with – heart and
gastrointestinal defects, deafness*

Pierre Robin

Retrognathia (abnormal jaw or
maxilla)
Micrognathia (small lower jaw)
Glossoptosis (tongue falls back)
Natal teeth
*Associated with – difficulty breathing;
cleft, holed or high arched palate;
a second syndrome (e.g. FAS)*

Poland

Concave chest (absent or reduced
muscle)
Abnormal or short ribs
Nipple abnormalities
Short radius and ulna on affected
side
Abnormal hand on same side –
webbed or fused fingers
*Associated with – Sprengel deformity,
facial paralysis, leukaemia,
non-Hodgkin's lymphoma*

Prader–Willi

Hypotonia
Weak reflexes
Poor suck reflex/poor feeder
Almond-shaped eyes
Small hands and feet
Weak cry
Thin upper lip
Down-turned mouth
Hypogonadism
Scoliosis
*Associated with – one or more
undescended testis*

Turner

Low birth weight
Females only
Swollen hands
Thick neck tissue
*Associated with – infertility, heart and
kidney abnormalities*

Treacher Collins

Absent malar bones
Downward slanting eyes
Micrognathia
Abnormal ears
*Associated with – cleft palate,
respiratory problems*

Zellweger

Hypotonia
Wide-set eyes
Under-developed eyebrow ridges
Poor suck and swallow
Enlarged liver
Seizures
*Associated with – jaundice,
gastrointestinal bleeding*

49 Scenarios

In all the scenario situations highlighted here, you should refer to your local NHS Trust policy, national guidance and the available contemporary literature. Analysis and critical exploration of your sources of evidence and the incorporation of parental needs should be considered.

1 A baby is found to have bilateral undescended testes. Please discuss the significance of this and appropriate management. Would there have been a different management pathway in the event of unilateral undescended testis?

2 During the NIPE examination, the baby is found to have a positive screen when conducting the Barlow's manoeuvre. Why is this significant and how should this be managed?

3 What information would you give parents regarding 'safer-sleeping' and 'tummy time'?

4 Why is it important for parents to be aware that their baby should be able to fixate and follow an object/light with his/her eyes and have some understanding of the extent of their baby's sight during the neonatal period?

5 How many reflexes can be seen or provoked in the newborn baby and why are they important?

6 The baby's mother asks you what to use to moisturise her newborn son's skin as he is a bit 'dry and flaky'. What information might you give her?

7 Prior to auscultating the baby's heart, what do the parents need to know?

8 You are about to conduct a NIPE on a 10-hour-old newborn baby when you notice that the baby appears to be jaundiced. What information would you give the parents and what action might you take and why?

9 The baby you have examined has talipes. Discuss predisposing factors and the treatment for unilateral and bilateral talipes.

10 What is the current management in the event of the mother having group B streptococcus and how would you recognise if her baby showed signs of infection?

11 Hyperpigmented macules are not an unusual occurrence. What information would you give the parents in relation to this birthmark and what would you document and why?

12 What significance is attached to finding meconium stained amniotic fluid (MSAF) during labour/birth and how might this knowledge affect your management?

13 Discuss the reasons why a baby may appear jittery or have tremors?

14 How does knowledge of the energy triangle assist when managing neonatal hypothermia?

15 When examining a baby, you notice that the legs are consistently held at approximately a 90 degree verticle angle to his/her body. What is the significance of this and what actions may you need to take?

16 Why might you suspect hypoglycaemia in a newborn baby and what are the risk factors and care practices that might make an impact on this condition?

17 How might you recognise a subaponeurotic (or subgaleal) haemorrhage and why is early recognition important?

18 A mother has given birth to a female baby, 3 hours ago and now wants to go home. What is the current thinking about the timing of the NIPE? What information would you give the parents and why?

19 What is the rationale and information you should give parents about the use of car seats and baby slings?

20 You find a small white 'blister' on the tip of the penis of a 9-hour-old newborn baby is this significant?

Crosswords and multiple choice questions

Crosswords

Crossword 1

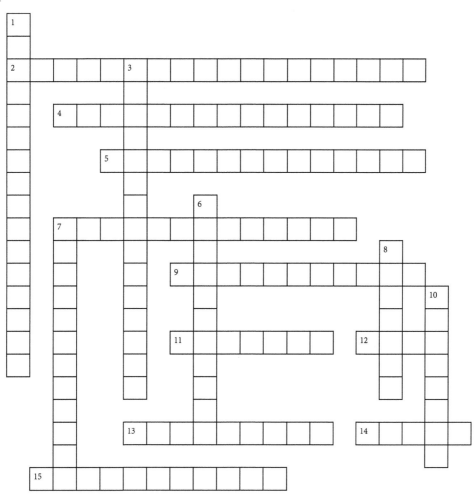

Across

2 The slightly blood-stained vaginal loss in the neonate [18]
4 What type of haemorrhage caused by the pressure of labour can be seen in the sclera of the neonatal eye? [15]
5 Small, white spots or cysts found on the soft palate or penis of the neonate [8,6]
7 The result of low blood sugar [13]
9 When the hand has more than five digits [11]
11 A foot deformity that can be classed as 'positional' or 'fixed' [7]
12 Reflex where the hands/arms extend outwards and then make a slight movement inwards [4]
13 A genetic abnormality that may portray one palmar crease [7,2]
14 The scoring system used to assess neonatal well-being soon after birth [5]
15 A cold baby is suffering from — [11]

Down

1 Soft oedematous patch found on the neonatal head after birth [5,11]
3 What is the head circumference measurement called? [8-7]
6 When the urethral opening is found on the underside of the penis [11]
7 NIPE highlights four particular elements of the physical examination of the newborn – cardiac, eyes, testes. What is the fourth area? [3,9]
8 What does the brain need to work effectively? [7]
10 What does the neonate metabolise for glucose/heat production? [5,3]

Physical Examination of the Newborn at a Glance, First Edition. Denise (Dee) Campbell and Lyn Dolby.
© 2018 John Wiley & Sons, Ltd. Published 2018 by John Wiley & Sons, Ltd.

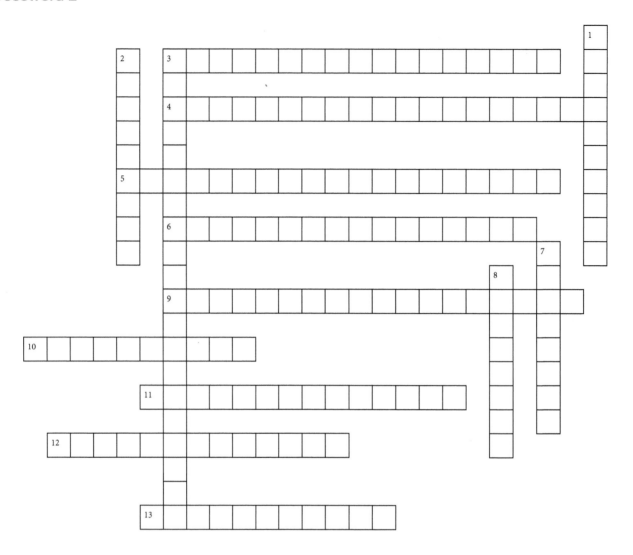

Across

3 Remnant of the ductus venosus [10,7]

4 A leading cause of bacterial sepsis in term neonates [5,1,13]

5 Meconium aspiration can cause this [8,11]

6 The most common platelet disorder [16]

9 A leading cause of pathological jaundice during the first 24 hours [1,1,1,15]

10 Deficiency of this substance can contribute to respiratory distress syndrome [10]

11 Another term for undescended testis [14]

12 What is the medical term for tongue tie? [13]

13 Defect in umbilicus with herniation of abdominal contents [11]

Down

1 Condition in which the urethra opens on the dorsal aspect of the penis [10]

2 This causes part of the male anatomy to light up like a light bulb [9]

3 Remnant of the ductus arteriosus [10,10]

7 A clouding of the lens of the eye [8]

8 A defect in melanin production that produces a lack of pigment [8]

Multiple choice questions

The following MCQs provide a self-test quiz for you to test your knowledge and understanding.

1 **Where is the lambda situated?**
   A At the junction of the parietal and frontal bones
   B At the junction of the parietal and occipital bones
   C At the junction of the occipital and frontal bones
   D At the junction of the parietal and temporal bones

2 **Acrocyanosis is the term used for which of the following states?**
   A Transient mottling of the skin
   B Neonatal hands and feet remain blue after birth
   C Slight blueness surrounding the neonatal mouth
   D Blue mucous membranes

3 **Occasionally, a neonate demonstrates a clear demarcated area of redness and an area of paleness that divides the neonate from head to abdomen. What is this called?**
   A Plethora
   B Cutis marmarata
   C Harlequin colour change
   D Acrocyanosis

4 **If polyhydramnios presents during pregnancy, which of the following conditions is the baby at risk of?**
   A Oesophageal atresia
   B Abdominal gastritis
   C Prune belly syndrome
   D Renal agenesis

5 **Which one of the following gives the measurement for the posterior fontanelle?**
   A 1 × 1 cm
   B 3.4 × 1.5 cm
   C 6.1 × 3 cm
   D 3 × 3 cm

6 **Physiological jaundice is caused by which of the following?**
   A Infection
   B ABO incompatability
   C Natural breakdown of excess red blood cells
   D Rhesus isoimmunisation

7 **A normal newborn rash is often seen in the neonate during the first week of life. What is the medical term for this type of rash?**
   A Vernix caseosa
   B Erythema toxicum neonatorum
   C Naevus flammeus
   D None of the above

8 **In the event of undescended testis, there is an increased risk of which of the following?**
   A Prune belly syndrome
   B Hypospadias
   C Malignancy
   D Neuroblastoma

9 **Early signs of neonatal infection are often subtle. Which of the following is generally considered to be a later sign of infection?**
   A Apnoea
   B Tachypnoea
   C Irritability
   D Convulsions

10 **Which of the following is NOT considered to be a neonatal neurological alarm signal?**
   A Persistent irritability
   B Bilateral and equal Moro reflex
   C Floppiness/severe generalised hypotonia
   D Abnormal cry

11 **Which of the following reflexes is NOT seen at birth but is normally fully developed by 6–8 months of age?**
   A Moro reflex
   B Symmetric tonic neck reflex
   C Placing and stepping
   D Rooting and suckling

12 **Which of the following is a common sign of intracranial haemorrhage in the term neonate?**
   A Normal neurological behaviour
   B Seizures
   C Pale skin
   D None of the above

13 **Which of the following is a classic sign of Erb's palsy following a brachial plexus injury at birth?**
   A Torticollis
   B Flexed arms
   C 'Waiter's tip' posture
   D None of the above

14 **Macrocephaly is defined as which of the following?**
   A Soft skull bones
   B Distortion of the cranium
   C Excessively large head
   D Enlarged head caused by excess cerebrospinal fluid

15 **Macroglossia is defined as which of the following?**
   A Large protruding tongue
   B Small tongue
   C Bright red tongue
   D None of the above

16 **Micrognathia is defined as which of the following?**
   A Abnormally large chin
   B Abnormally small chin
   C Webbing of the neck
   D None of the above

17 **Chordee is defined as which of the following?**
   A Abnormally long penis
   B Masculine genitals
   C Larger than average testes
   D Ventral curvature of the penis

Crosswords and multiple choice answers

Crosswords

Crossword 1

Across

2 PSEUDOMENSTRUATION – the slightly blood-stained vaginal loss in the neonate

4 SUBCONJUNCTIVAL – haemorrhage caused by the pressure of labour that can be visible in the sclera of the neonatal eye

5 EPSTEINS PEARLS – small, white spots or cysts found on the soft palate or penis of the neonate

7 HYPOGLYCAEMIA – the result of low blood sugar

9 POLYDACTYLY – when the hand has more than five digits

11 TALIPES – a foot deformity that can be classed as 'positional' or 'fixed'

12 MORO – reflex in which the hands/arms extend outwards and then make a slight movement inwards

13 TRISOMY 21 – a genetic abnormality that may portray a number of signs such as 'one palmar crease, and is diagnosed via DNA testing

14 APGAR – the scoring system used to assess neonatal wellbeing soon after birth

15 HYPOTHERMIA – see chapter on thermoregulation

Down

1 CAPUT SUCCEDANEUM – soft oedematous patch found on the neonatal head after birth

3 OCCIPITO-FRONTAL – head circumference measurement

6 HYPOSPADIAS – when the urethral opening is found on the underside of the penis

7 HIP STABILITY – NIPE elements for the physical examination of the newborn are cardiac, eyes, testes and hips, but obviously also includes the systematic examination of the rest of the body and reflexes

8 GLUCOSE – the brain runs on this

10 BROWN FAT – the neonate can metabolise this for glucose/heat production

Crossword 2

Across

3 LIGAMENTUM VENOSUM – remnant of the ductus venosus

4 GROUP B STREPTOCOCCUS – a leading cause of bacterial sepsis in term neonates

5 CHEMICAL PNEUMONITIS – meconium aspiration can cause this

6 THROMBOCYTOPENIA – the most common platelet disorder

9 A B O INCOMPATIBILITY – a leading cause of pathological jaundice during the first 24 hours

10 SURFACTANT – deficiency of this substance can contribute to respiratory distress syndrome

11 CRYPTORCHIDISM – another term for undescended testis

12 ANKYLOGLOSSIA – the medical term for tongue tie

13 OMPHALOCELE – defect in umbilicus with herniation of abdominal contents

Down

1 EPISPADIAS – condition in which the urethra opens on the dorsal aspect of the penis

2 HYDROCELE – causes part of the male anatomy to light up like a light bulb

3 LIGAMENTUM ARTERIOSUM – remnant of the ductus arteriosus

7 CATARACT – a clouding in the lens of the eye

8 ALBINISM – a defect in melanin production that produces a lack of pigment

Multiple choice answers

The following MCQs provide a self-test quiz for you to test your knowledge and understanding.

1 **Where is the lambda situated?**
The correct answer is B.

2 **Acrocyanosis is the term used for which of the following states?**
The correct answer is B.

3 **Occasionally, a neonate demonstrates a clear demarcated area of redness and an area of paleness that divides the neonate from head to abdomen. What is this called?**
The correct answer is C.

4 **If polyhydramnios presents during pregnancy, which of the following conditions is the baby at risk of?**
The correct answer is A.

5 **Which one of the following gives the measurement for the posterior fontanelle?**
The correct answer is A.

6 **Physiological jaundice is caused by which of the following?**
The correct answer is C.

7 **A normal newborn rash is often seen in the neonate during the first week of life. What is the medical term for this type of rash?**
The correct answer is B.

8 **In the event of undescended testis, there is an increased risk of which of the following?**
The correct answer is C.

9 **Early signs of neonatal infection are often subtle. Which of the following is generally considered to be a later sign of infection?**
The correct answer is D.

10 **Which of the following is NOT considered to be a neonatal neurological alarm signal?**
The correct answer is B.

11 **Which of the following reflexes is NOT seen at birth but is normally fully developed by 6–8 months of age?**
The correct answer is B.

12 **Which of the following is a common sign of intracranial haemorrhage in the term neonate?**
The correct answer is C.

13 **Which of the following is a classic sign of Erb's palsy following a brachial plexus injury at birth?**
The correct answer is C.

14 **Macrocephaly is defined as which of the following?**
The correct answer is C.

15 **Macroglossia is defined as which of the following?**
The correct answer is A.

16 **Micrognathia is defined as which of the following?**
The correct answer is B.

17 **Chordee is defined as which of the following?**
The correct answer is D.

References

Abdelrahman W and Abdelmageed A. (2014) Medical record keeping: Clarity, accuracy, and timeliness are essential. UK. British Medical Journal Careers. http://careers.bmj.com/careers/advice/Medical_record_keeping%3A_clarity%2C_accuracy%2C_and_timeliness_are_essential (accessed 12 October 2017).

Aylott M. (2006) The neonatal energy triangle. Part 1: Metabolic adaptation. *Paediatric Nursing*, **18** (6), 38–42.

Birthmark Unit. (2012) *Port Wine Stains: Information For Families*. Birthmark Unit, Great Ormond Street, London.

Black J and Rose P. (2000) Temperature measurement in the preterm infant: a literature review. *Journal of Neonatal Nursing*, **6** (1), 28–32.

Brazelton T and Nugent K. (2011) *Clinics in Developmental Medicine no. 190: The Neonatal Behavioural Assessment Scale* (4th edn). MacKeith Press, London.

British Association of Perinatal Medicine (2015) Newborn Early Warning Trigger and Track (NEWTT) chart: A Framework for Practice. British Association of Perinatal Medicine. https://www.bapm.org/sites/default/files/files/NEWTT%20framework%20final.pdf (accessed 12 October 2017).

British Association of Perinatal Medicine (BAPM) (2017) Identification and Management of Neonatal Hypoglycaemia in the Full Term Infant. A Framework for Practice. BAPM. https://www.bapm.org/resources/identification-and-management-neonatal-hypoglycaemia-full-term-infant-%E2%80%93-framework-practice (accessed 12 October 2017).

Brozansky BS, Riley MM and Bogen DL. (2012) Neonatology, in *Atlas of Pediatric Diagnosis* (6th edn) (eds BJ Zitelli, SC McIntire and AJ Nowalk). Elsevier Saunders, Philadelphia.

Centers of Disease Control and Prevention (CDC) (2015) Birth Defects. Facts about Cleft Lip and Cleft Palate. http://www.cdc.gov/ncbddd/birthdefects/cleftlip.html (accessed 12 October 2017).

Children Act 2004. Chapter 31. HMSO, London. http://www.legislation.gov.uk/ukpga/2004/31/pdfs/ukpga_20040031_en.pdf (accessed 12 October 2017).

Clarke M. (2013) Clinical update: understanding jaundice in the breastfed infant. *Community Practitioner*, **86** (6), 42–44.

Colditz M, Lai M, Cartwright D and Colditz P. (2014) Subgaleal haemorrhage in the newborn: A call for early diagnosis and aggressive management. *Journal of Paediatrics and Child Health*, **51** (2), 140–146.

Cooke A, Cork MJ, Victor S, *et al.* (2015) Olive oil, sunflower oil or no oil for baby dry skin or massage: a pilot, assessor-blinded, randomized controlled trial (Oil in Baby SkincaRE [OBSeRvE] Study). *Acta Dermato-Venereologica*, **96** (3), 1–9. doi:10.2340/00015555-2279

Cross H. (2013) Differential diagnosis of epileptic seizures in infancy including the neonatal period. *Seminars in Fetal and Neonatal Medicine*, **18** (4), 192–195.

Crozier K and Macdonald S. (2010) Effective skin-care regimes for term newborn infants: A structured literature review. *Evidence Based Midwifery*, **8** (4), 128–135.

General Medical Council (2012) Protecting children and young people, the responsibilities of all doctors. General Medical Council, UK. http://www.gmc-uk.org/static/documents/content/Protecting_children_and_young_people_-_English_1015.pdf (accessed 12 October 2017).

Godley DR. (2013) Assessment, diagnosis, and treatment of developmental dysplasia of the hip. *JAAPA*, **26** (3), 54–58.

Green TL. (2012) Black and immigrant: Exploring the effects of ethnicity and foreign-born status on infant health. A project of the Migration Policy Institute's National Center on Immigration Integration Policy. https://www.migrationpolicy.org/research/CBI-infant-health (accessed 12 October 2017).

Greig C. (1999) Trauma during birth, haemorrhage and convulsions, in *Myles Textbook for Midwives* (eds VR Bennett and LK Brown). Churchill Livingstone, London. pp. 777–793.

Haas DM, Sischy AC, McCullough W and Simsiman AJ. (2011) Maternal ethnicity influences on neonatal respiratory outcomes after antenatal corticosteroid use for anticipated preterm delivery. *Journal of Maternal and Fetal Neonatal Medicine*, **24** (3), 516–520. doi: 10.3109/14767058.2010.506228

Harrison S, Buttner P and Nowak M. (2005) Maternal beliefs about the reputed therapeutic uses of sun exposure in infancy and the postpartum period. *Australian Midwifery Journal*, **18** (2), 22–28.

Hart AR, Pilling EL and Alix JJP. (2015) Neonatal seizures – part 1: Not everything that jerks, stiffens and shakes is a fit. *Archives of Disease in Childhood. Education and Practice Edition*, **100**, 170–175. doi:10.1136/archdischild-2014-306385

Hautemaniere A, Cunat L, Diguio N, *et al.* (2010) Factors determining poor practice in alcoholic hand gel rub technique in hospital workers. *Journal of Infection and Public Health*, **3** (1), 25–34.

Hawdon J. (2015) Postnatal metabolic adaptation and neonatal hypoglycaemia. *Paediatrics and Child Health*, **26** (4), 135–139.

Hawdon JM, Beer J, Sharp D, *et al.* (2017) Neonatal hypoglycaemia: learning from claims. *Archives of Disease in Childhood. Fetal Neonatal Edition*, **102** (2), F110–F115.

Horimukai K. (2014) Application of moisturizer to neonates prevents development of atopic dermatitis. *J Allergy Clin Immunol*, **134** (4), 824–830.

Illingworth R. (1987) *The Development of the Infant and Young Child: Normal and Abnormal*. Churchill Livingstone, Edinburgh.

Irvine A, Hoeger P and Yan A. (eds) (2011) *Harper's Textbook of Pediatric Dermatology* (3rd edn). Blackwell Publishing, Oxford.

Jackson A. (2008) Time to review newborn skin care. *Infant*, **4** (5), 168–171.

Kramer LI. (1969) Advancement of dermal icterus in the jaundiced newborn. *American Journal of Diseases of Children*, **118**, 454–458.

Lissauer T and Fanaroff AA. (2011) *Neonatology at a Glance* (2nd edn). Wiley Blackwell, Oxford.

Lissauer T, Fanaroff A and Miall L. (2014) *Neonatology at a Glance* (3rd edn). Wiley Blackwell, Oxford.

Louis GB, Grewal J, Albert P, *et al.* (2015) Racial/ethnic differences in fetal growth: The NICHD fetal growth studies.

American Journal of Obstetrics and Gynaecology, **212** (1), 536. doi.org/10.1016/j.ajog.2014.10.098

Mace J and Paton R. (2015) Neonatal clinical screening of the hip in the diagnosis of developmental dysplasia of the hip: a 15-year prospective longitudinal observational study. *Bone Joint Journal*, **97-B** (2), 265–269.

McLaughlin M, O'Connor N and Ham P. (2008) Newborn skin. Part II: Birthmarks. *American Family Physician*, **77** (1), 56–60.

Midwifery 2020 (2010). *Midwifery 2020 Programme Core Role of the Midwife Workstream Final Report.* Midwifery 2020, London.

National Institute for Health and Care Excellence (NICE) (2012a) Social and emotional wellbeing – early years. (PH40) Manchester: NICE. https://www.nice.org.uk/guidance/ph40/chapter/glossary#vulnerable-children (accessed 12 October 2017).

National Institute for Health and Care Excellence (NICE) (2012b) Healthcare-associated infections: prevention and control in primary and community care. Clinical guideline (CG 139). http://www.nice.org.uk/guidance/cg139 (accessed 12 October 2017).

National Institute for Health and Care Excellence (NICE) (2014) Intrapartum care for healthy women and babies. Clinical guideline (CG 190). http://www.nice.org.uk/guidance/cg190 (accessed 12 October 2017).

National Institute for Health and Care Excellence (NICE) (2015) Postnatal care up to 8 weeks after birth. Clinical Guideline (CG 37). https://www.nice.org.uk/guidance/cg37 (accessed 12 October 2017).

National Institute for Health and Care Excellence (NICE) (2016) Neonatal jaundice: Assessment. Neonatal Pathways. Clinical guideline (CG 98). https://www.nice.org.uk/guidance/cg98 (accessed 12 October 2017).

Nursing and Midwifery Council (NMC) (2015) *The Code: Professional Standards of Practice and Behaviour for Nurses and Midwives.* NMC.

Public Health England (PHE) (2016a) Newborn and Infant Physical Examination Screening Programme Handbook 2016/2017. UK National Screening Committee. PHE publications gateway number: 2015772. https://www.gov.uk/government/publications/newborn-and-infant-physical-examination-programme-handbook (accessed 12 October 2107).

Public Health England (PHE) (2016b) Newborn and Infant Physical Examination Screening Programme Standards 2016/2017. UK National Screening Committee. PHE publications gateway number: 2015772. https://www.gov.uk/government/publications/newborn-and-infant-physical-examination-screening-standards (accessed 12 October 2107).

Public Health England (PHE) (2016c) Guidelines for Newborn Blood Spot Sampling. UK National Screening Committee. PHE publications gateway number: 2015750. https://www.gov.uk/government/uploads/system/uploads/attachment_data/file/511688/Guidelines_for_Newborn_Blood_Spot_Sampling_January_2016.pdf (accessed 12 October 2017).

Public Health England (PHE) (2017) Pulse Oximetry Pilot Trial 2015. UK NSC Blog. https://phescreening.blog.gov.uk/2017/01/10/newborn-pulse-oximetry-screening-pilot-update/ (accessed 12 October 2017).

Queensland Maternity and Neonatal Clinical Guidelines Programme (2012) Neonatal Jaundice. Clinical Guideline. Queensland Government. https://www.health.qld.gov.au/__data/assets/pdf_file/0018/142038/g_jaundice.pdf (accessed 12 October 2017).

Resuscitation Council (UK) (2015) Resuscitation and support of transition of babies at birth. Chapter 7: Explanatory notes.

https://www.resus.org.uk/resuscitation-guidelines/resuscitation-and-support-of-transition-of-babies-at-birth/ (accessed 12 October 2017).

Roposch A, Protopapa E, Cortina-Borja M. (2014) Weighted diagnostic criteria for developmental dysplasia of the hip. *Journal of Pediatrics*, **165** (6), 1236–1240.

Rosendahl K, Dezateux C, Fosse K, *et al.* (2010) Immediate treatment versus sonographic surveillance for mild hip dysplasia in newborns. *Pediatrics*, **125** (1), 9–16.

Royal College of Midwives (RCM) (2014) Maternal mental health: Improving emotional wellbeing in postnatal care. https://www.rcm.org.uk/sites/default/files/Pressure%20Points%20-%20Mental%20Health%20-%20Final_0.pdf (accessed 12 October 2017).

Royal College of Obstetricians and Gynaecologists (RCOG) (2017) Maternal Mental Health – Women's Voices. https://www.rcog.org.uk/globalassets/documents/patients/information/maternalmental-healthwomens-voices.pdf (accessed 12 October 2017).

Ruth VA. (2007) Neonatal surgical disorders of the head, eyes, nose and throat, in *Neonatal Surgical Procedures. A Guide for care and Management* (eds DB Longobucco and VA Ruth). NICU Ink Book Publishers, California. pp. 1–58.

Rychik J, Donaghue D, Levy S, *et al.* (2013) Maternal psychological stress after prenatal diagnosis of congenital heart disease. *Journal of Pediatrics*, **162** (2), 302–307. doi.org/10.1016/j.jpeds.2012.07.023

Scott B. (2016) What is an oral cyst? WiseGEEK. http://www.wisegeekhealth.com/what-is-an-oral-cyst.htm (accessed 12 October 2017).

Sinha S, Miall L and Jardin L. (2012) *Essential Neonatal Medicine* (5th edn). Wiley Blackwell, Oxford.

Sletner L, Nakstad B, Yajnik CS, *et al.* (2013) Ethnic differences in neonatal body composition in a multi-ethnic population and the impact of parental factors: A population-based cohort study. *PLoS ONE*, **8** (8), e73058. doi:10.1371/journal.pone.0073058

Solak, S. (2016) Prevalence of congenital cutaneous anomalies in 1000 newborns and a review of the literature. *American Journal of Perinatology*, **33** (1), 79–83.

Sollai S, Dani C, Berti E, *et al.* (2016) Performance of a non-contact infrared thermometer in healthy newborns. *British Medical Journal*, BMJ Open. http://bmjopen.bmj.com/content/6/3/e008695.full.pdf+html (accessed 12 October 2017).

Sotiriadis A, Papatheodorou S, Eleftheriades M and Makrydimas G. (2013) Nuchal translucency and major congenital heart defects in fetuses with normal karyotype: A meta-analysis. *Ultrasound in Obstetrics and Gynecology*, **42** (4), 383–389.

Stables D and Rankin J. (2010) *Physiology in Childbearing: With Anatomy and Related Biosciences* (3rd edn). Bailliere Tindall.

Stringer MD, Sugarman I and Smyth AG. (2005) Congenital defects and surgical problems, in *Roberton's Textbook of Neonatology* (4th edn). (ed. JM Rennie). Elsevier Churchill Livingstone, Philadelphia, PA.

Sutton G, Wood S, Feirn R, Minchom S, Parker G and Sirimanna T. (2012) *Newborn Hearing Screening and Assessment: Guidelines for Surveillance and Audiological Referral of Infants and Children Following the Newborn Hearing Screen.* Version 5.1. June. NHSP Clinical Group.

Swetman GL, Lee D and Benjamin L. (2011) Nevi in the newborn. *Neoreviews*, **12** (4), e207–215.

Swingler M, Perry N, Bell M and Calkin S. (2017) Maternal behavior predicts infant neurophysiological and behavioral attention processes in the first year. *Developmental Psychology*, **53** (1), 13–27.

Tappero EP. (2009) Musculoskeletal system assessment, in *Physical Assessment of the Newborn: A Comprehensive Approach to the Art of Physical Examination* (eds EP Tappero and ME Honeyfield). NICUINK Book Publishers, California. pp 133–157.

Thomas RK. (2015) *Practical Medical Procedures at a Glance*. Wiley Blackwell, Oxford.

Torjesen I. (2013) Swaddling increases babies risk of hip abnormalities. *British Medical Journal*, **347**, f6499.

United Kingdom Department of Education (2015a) *Working Together to Safeguard Children: A Guide to Inter-Agency Working to Safeguard and Promote the Welfare of Children*. HMSO, London.

United Kingdom Department of Education (2015b) The Children Act 1989: Guidance and Regulations Volume 2: Care Planning, Placement and Case Review. https://www.gov.uk/government/uploads/system/uploads/attachment_data/file/441643/Children_Act_Guidance_2015.pdf (accessed 12 October 2017).

Vasudevan C and Levene M. (2013) Epidemiology and aetiology of neonatal seizures. *Seminars in Fetal and Neonatal Medicine*, **18** (4), 185–191. doi.org/10.1016/j.siny.2013.04.003

Villar J, Papageorghiou AT, Pang R, *et al.* (2014) The likeness of fetal growth and newborn size across non-isolated populations in the INTERGROWTH-21st Project: the Fetal Growth Longitudinal Study and Newborn Cross-Sectional Study for the International Fetal and Newborn Growth Consortium for the 21st Century (INTERGROWTH-21st) *The Lancet. Diabetes and Endocrinology*, **2** (10), 781–792.

Waldron S and Mackinnon R. (2007) Neonatal thermoregulation. *Infant*, **3** (3), 101–104.

Walker K, Vangipuram SD and Kalra K. (2014) Congenital pseudoarthrosis of the clavicle: A diagnostic challenge. *Global Paediatric Health*, **Jan-Dec**, 1–3.

Wall L, Mills J, Leveno K, *et al.* (2014) Incidence and prognosis of neonatal brachial plexus palsy with and without clavicle fractures. *Obstetrics and Gynecology*, **123** (6), 1288–93. doi:10.1097/AOG.0000000000000207

Watkins J. (2016) Common skin complaints in neonates. *British Journal of Midwifery*, **24** (1), 12–16.

Williams J. (2012) The recognition and management of isolated cleft palate. *Community Practice*, **85**, 28–31.

Woodacre T, Dhadwal A, Ball T, Edwards C, Cox P. (2014) The costs of late detection of developmental dysplasia of the hip. *Journal of Children's Orthopaedics*, **8** (4), 325–332.

World Health Organization (WHO) (2007) *Child Growth Standards: Head circumference-for-age, arm circumference-for-age, triceps skin fold-for-age and, subscapular skin fold-for age: methods and development*. WHO, Geneva.

World Health Organization (WHO) (2009) *Guidelines on Hand Hygiene in Health Care*. WHO, Geneva. http://apps.who.int/iris/bitstream/10665/44102/1/9789241597906_eng.pdf (accessed 12 October 2017).

Useful websites

Department of Health, Childhood Immunisation Schedule: https://www.gov.uk/government/publications/routine-childhood-immunisation-schedule

International Hip Dysplasia Institute: http://hipdysplasia.org/

IT NIPE SMART: https://cpdscreening.phe.org.uk/nipe-smart#fileid14098

Lullaby Trust – Research and information on Sudden Infant Death syndrome: www.lullabytrust.org.uk

NHS England. Patient safety expert groups and steering group: https://www.england.nhs.uk/patientsafety/patient-safety-groups/

Personal Child Health Record (PCHR): http://www.healthforallchildren.com/the-pchr/

Useful e-learning resources

Newborn Blood Spot Screening: https://cpdscreening.phe.org.uk/bloodspot-elearning

Newborn and Infant Physiological Examination: https://cpdscreening.phe.org.uk/nipe-elearning

Index

Locators in *italic* refer to figures/tables/boxes